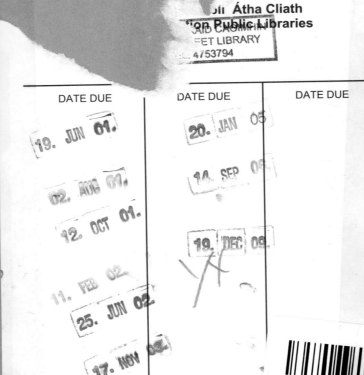

Leslie Kenton's
HEALING HERBS

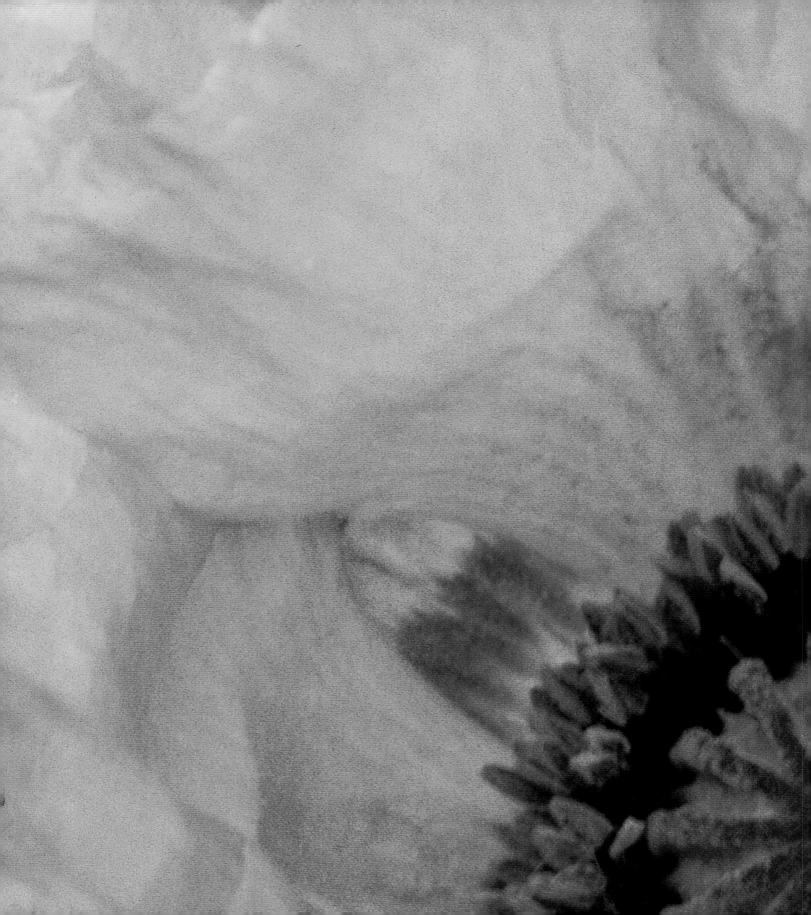

Leslie Kenton's
HEALING HERBS

Energy, health and great looks – right here, right now

Ebury Press
London

The material in this book is intended for information purposes only. None of the suggestions are meant to be prescriptive and no one can guarantee the curative effects of any of the herbs listed. Anything can be dangerous if used incorrectly. Neither I nor the publisher can accept responsibility for injuries or illness arising out of a failure by a reader to correctly follow any of the directions contained in this book, or to take medical advice. Any attempt to treat a medical condition – and any treatment of children at all – should always come under the direction of a competent professional. Preferably this should be one who is familiar with herbal medicine, naturopathic techniques and nutrition.

If you are pregnant, unless you get the OK from your doctor, do not take herbs at all, except in the form of simple gentle herb teas like peppermint or ginger to calm an upset stomach, or camomile for sleep. Some herbs can increase the risk of miscarriage. So steer clear of barberry root bark, cascara sagrada, Chinese angelica, feverfew, juniper berries, mayapple, mugwort, pokeroot, pennyroyal, rue, senna, southernwood, tansey, thuja and wormwood. I would also steer clear of coffee – studies show that even the caffeine in one or two cups of brewed coffee drunk each day may double the risk of miscarriage and don't take more alcohol than the occasional glass of very good quality wine.

I have no commercial interest in any product, treatment or organization mentioned in this book. However, I have long sought to learn more about whatever can help us to live at a high level of energy, intelligence and creativity. For it is my belief that the more each one of us is able to re-establish harmony within ourselves and with our environment, the better equipped we shall be to wrestle with the challenges now facing our planet.

Leslie Kenton. Pembrokeshire, 2000

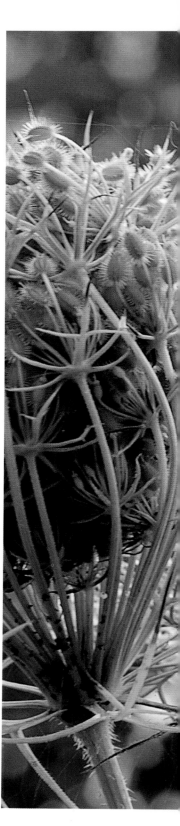

for Lada

whose beauty delights me …

whose awareness of the sacred enriches my life

First published in Great Britain in 2000

1 3 5 7 9 10 8 6 4 2

First published by
Ebury Press, Random House, 20 Vauxhall Bridge Road, London SW1V 2SA

Random House Australia (Pty) Limited
20 Alfred Street, Milsons Point, Sydney, New South Wales 2061, Australia

Random House New Zealand Limited
18 Poland Road, Glenfield, Auckland 10, New Zealand

Random House South Africa (Pty) Limited
Endulini, 5A Jubilee Road, Parktown 2193, South Africa

The Random House Group Limited Reg. No. 954009

www.randomhouse.co.uk

A CIP catalogue record for this book is available from the British Library.

Photographer: Leslie Kenton
Editor: Emma Callery
Designer: Ruth Prentice

ISBN 0091868386

Papers used by Ebury Press are natural, recyclable products made from wood grown in sustainable forests.

Printed and bound in Singapore by Tien Wah Press

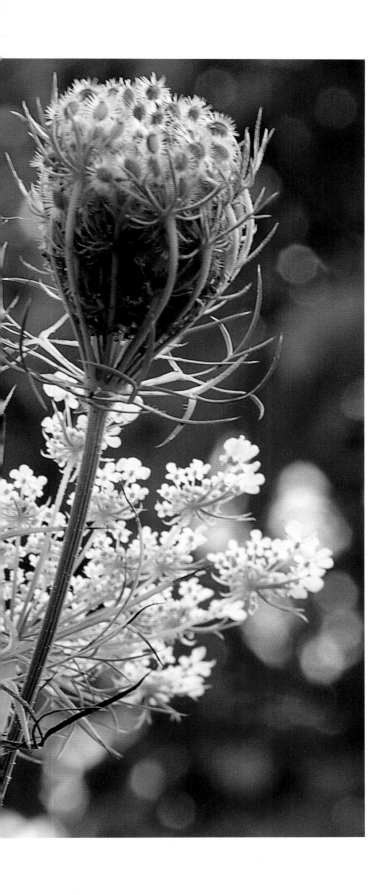

contents

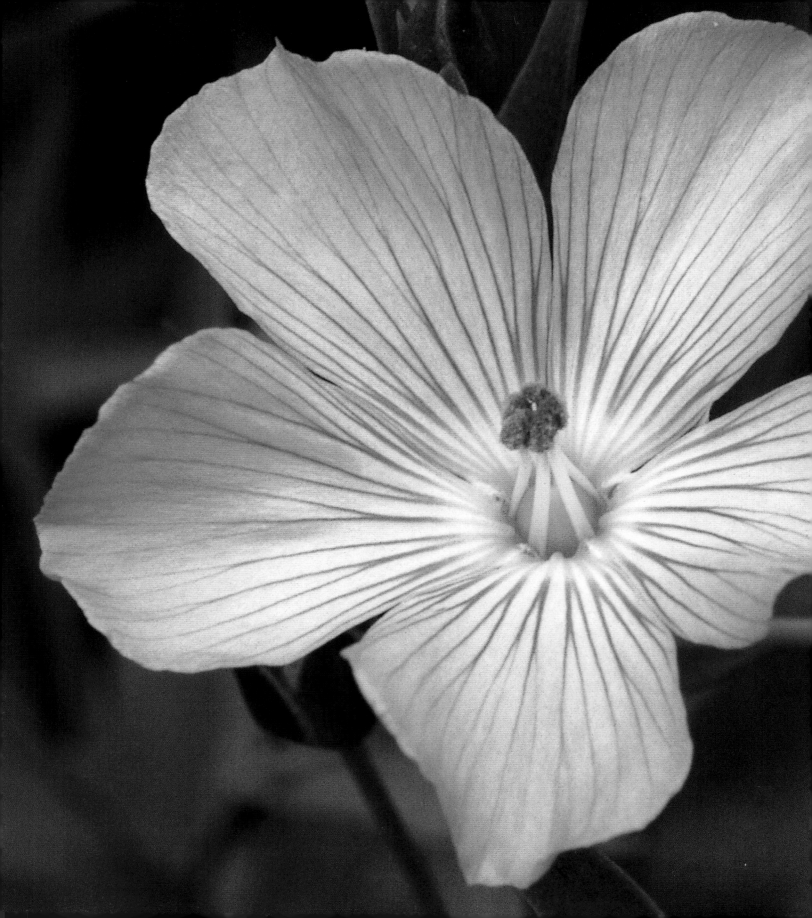

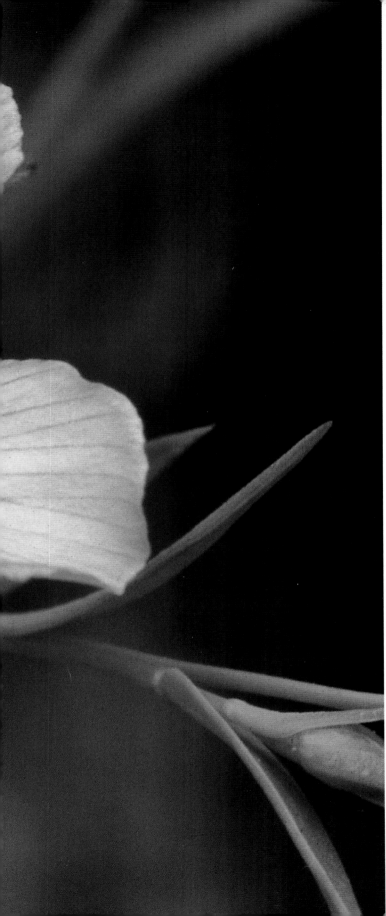

sheer pleasure

People everywhere are hungry for clear, practical, scientifically validated information about how to make use of herbs in their day-to-day lives. I too was once hungry for this kind of information. I discovered that working (and playing) with herbs did not need to be complex and confusing. It could be sheer pleasure. For me it was like walking down a path where a wonderful surprise is revealed at every turn.

◄ flax

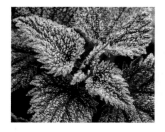

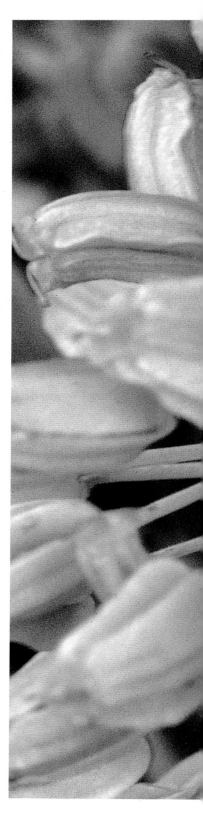

My passion for herbs began when I discovered the help they could bring me and my family. Simple plants like nettle or golden rod (*Solidago virgaurea*) have a natural cleansing and diuretic effect on the body. Travelling on airplanes my ankles would swell up. I discovered when I made a cup of golden rod or nettle tea that the swelling would vanish. Fascinated, I began to read about what herbs can do for the immune system. I started to experiment with plants like goldenseal and echinacea, burdock and shiitake mushrooms. My family took them whenever any of us threatened to come down with flu or a cold. And, provided we took them in time, a single herb or a combination of plants would usually clear the discomfort before the full force of illness hit.

A doctor friend, Gordon Latto, taught me that gargling with red sage and sticking a clove of garlic in its 'paper' shell in between the teeth and the inside of the mouth for a few hours a day would clear a sore throat and nip throat infections in the bud.

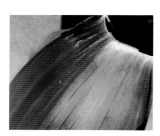

Another doctor, Philip Kilsby, taught me the power of detoxification for balancing the body and mind. Meanwhile, I developed a close friendship with Dr Dagmar Liechti von Brasch in Switzerland. Dr Liechti, niece of the famous Swiss physician Max Bircher Benner, continued to run the Bircher-Benner clinic for 40 years after his death. She taught me all about using herbs to handle women's problems from PMS to menopausal symptoms.

Before long I began to wonder just how many other remarkable things plants could do for us. I was lucky enough to spend time with the famous Russian scientist I.I. Brekhman, expert in adaptogenic herbs, whose research gained him the Lenin Prize for Science. From Brekhman I learned that special plants such as ginseng, astragalus and eleutherococcus – Siberian ginseng – strengthen a person's ability to resist illness. They also make it possible for us to work (and play) longer and harder without experiencing the negative effects of prolonged stress.

That was more than twenty years ago. Ever since I have used herbs and flowers, fresh raw juices and vegetables, water and tender loving care to help the body protect itself from illness, to heal a sickness when it strikes, to calm an agitated mind, to induce slumber when unable to sleep, to clear depression – even to intensify the whitish-blonde colour of my hair and care for my skin. I have also used herbs to decorate my house and to sanctify my working space.

capturing the beauty of herbs

My love affair with plants involved a fascination with their physical beauty too. I wanted to uncover the very essence of a plant's magic and share it with others. I became dissatisfied with the way herbs are so often portrayed in books. While nineteenth-century botanical drawings can be charming to look at, they often have a kind of sterility about them. They can look a bit like glass-encased butterflies stuck through with pins. Both

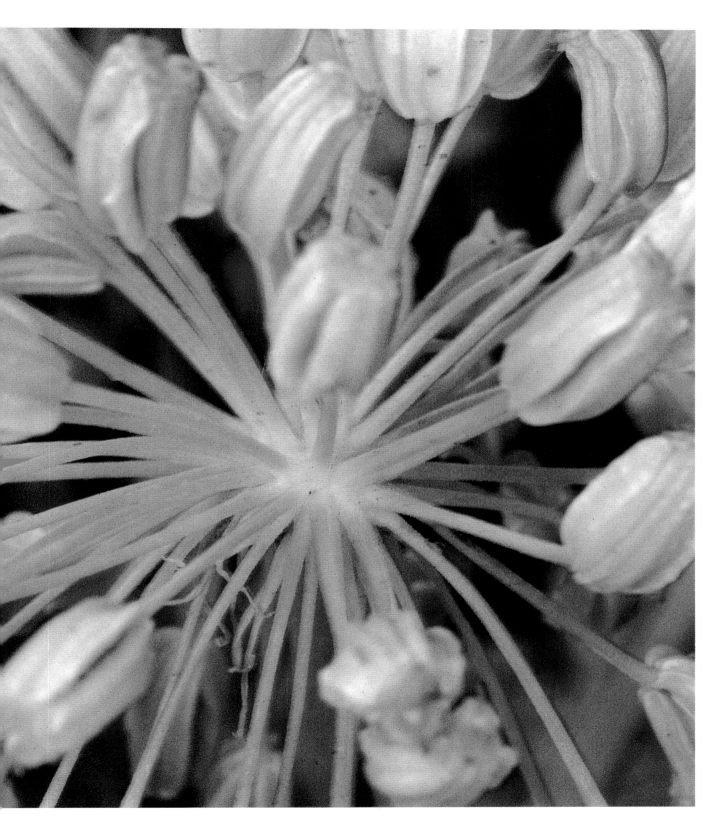

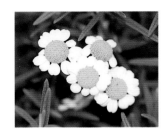

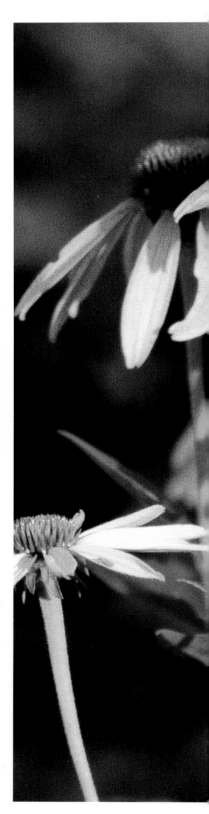

are indicative of a culture that viewed plants and animals as objects to be exploited by man. This was far from the sensuous relationship I experienced with these splendid living things, and far from how I wanted to share my experience of herbs with others.

So I began to experiment with macro-photography, where the camera is focused not only at the object but somehow into it. Most of the photographs in this book are either macro or micro – the closest photographs you can take without using a microscope. I had never taken such photographs before but I was determined to try. I discovered that photographing herbs much larger than life can indeed reveal more of their striking beauty. It also better reflects their essential nature, which we so often miss in our day-to-day interactions with plants. Almost before I realized what was happening, the private passion I had held for so long – which until then had focused on the practical, scientific and highly personal relationships I had with herbs – turned public. I knew I needed to find a way to share with others what I had discovered of the splendour and mystery of herbs – their power and their generosity. That is how this book came into being.

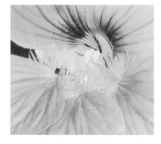

Within these pages you will find much about the chemistry of the most important power plants and cutting-edge clinical information that validates their traditional uses. All the way through I have attempted to put together practical, easy-to-use methods out of traditional repertoires gleaned from many years of travel throughout the world to learn more about plant lore and ancient practices. St John's wort (*Hypericum perforatum*), for instance, has been used for thousands of years as a nerve tonic, to ease anxiety and depression, enhance sleep and ease menopausal irritability. Recent research carried out in Germany shows that this herb can be as effective as Prozac in the treatment of depression and anxiety. Yet it comes without the side-effects of that drug. As a result, doctors there currently write more than 600,000 prescriptions for this plant every year.

Likewise, valerian, a remedy of choice for soothing stress and encouraging sleep, was shown in a recent Swiss study to ease insomnia in 89% of those who used it. And 44% of those participating in the trial claimed it brought 'perfect sleep' to them. Ginkgo has recently earned acclaim for its ability to treat the symptoms of Alzheimer's disease. Cranberry (traditionally used for bladder infections) has been shown to prevent bacteria sticking to the bladder walls so they can be flushed from the body. Meanwhile numerous studies show that ginseng helps protect the body from stress-caused damage.

reach out with your heart

Let your own romance with herbs begin as most do – tentatively. Have respect for plant life and maybe a touch of wonder. Try reaching out to plants to find out about them.

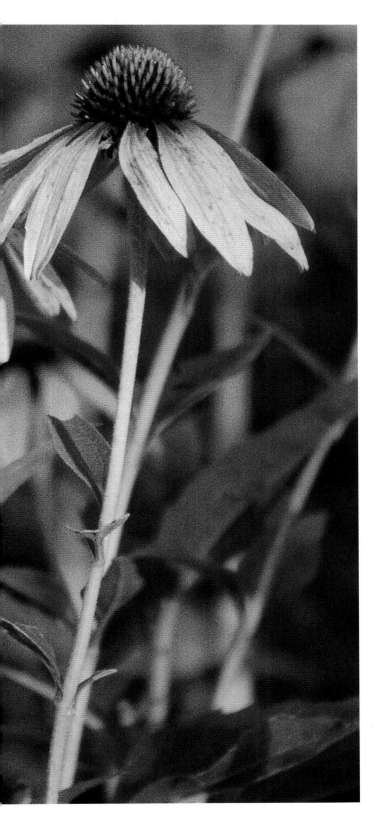

Be aware of how they smell, feel, and taste and how they affect you when you take them into your body. I grew herbs in my garden and in pots on my windowsills. I experimented with them by taking them myself and giving them to others. At first they were mostly those you use in cooking – rosemary, sage, marjoram, thyme and of course the mints. I loved these herbs and I looked for more and more varieties. Before long I became aware of the amazing energies that they carry. Pop a tiny mint plant into the soil in the early spring and by the next spring you will find it is rapidly taking over the garden. I began to look at herbs and plants and to ask what gave them this power for health and healing.

I read about plants and learned about them from women who knew far more than I, from doctors who had come to prefer plants to drugs, from lectures – and eventually from the Internet. By this time my romance with plants had escalated to a full-blown love affair. I wanted to celebrate their beauty and their power. I began trying to listen to these wonderful growing things and speaking to them the way native peoples do. I knew that this was how Dr Edward Bach discovered the remarkable healing and emotional balancing properties of flowers in the Welsh hills where he wandered – plants that are now world renowned as Dr Bach's Flower Remedies. Eventually I began to teach these techniques to others in my workshops. I discovered that every one of us has the capacity to communicate intuitively with plants. It is all a question of remembering how and then practising.

I hope that this book inspires you to develop your own personal relationship with plants – to explore for yourself the way to grow and gather herbs, to use them for beauty and to call on them for healing. I hope also to introduce you to an experience of the central core of man's traditional intimacy with plants which in our culture has been almost completely forgotten. For in addition to a plant's biochemical actions, in addition to its healing or beautifying properties, each plant – like each human being – has a highly specific personality. It is this sense of a personality that we come to know as we rediscover our ability to relate to plants intuitively. The more you explore a herb's personality, the more you allow its beauty and power to dazzle you, the greater are the gifts it brings you in return.

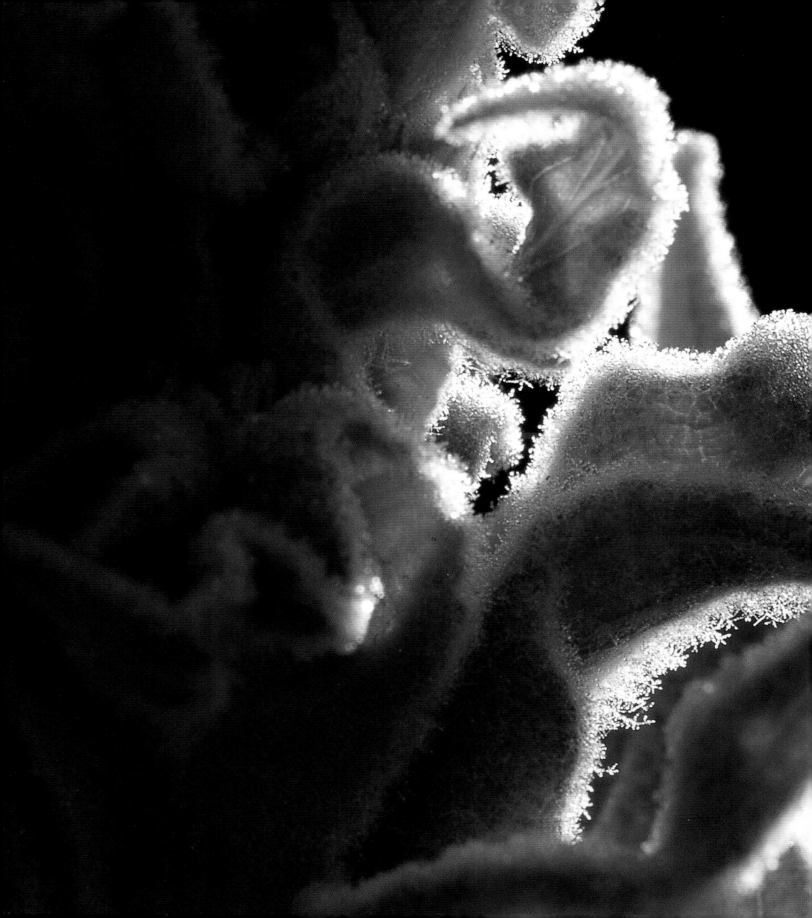

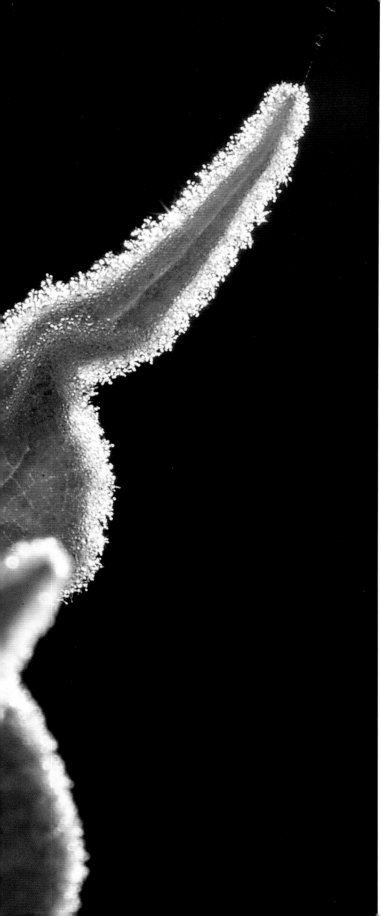

plant magic 1

For more than a million years our ancestors have lived with herbs. They cooked with them, healed with them, scented their bodies and sanctified their prayers with them. On a molecular level, the human body recognizes a herb when it is ingested. Discover the nature of a specific plant. It will enhance your life immeasurably. In a very real sense you can come to know a herb the way a woman knows her lover. When the spirit of a plant meets the spirit of a human, expect magic. You won't be disappointed.

◄ mullein

gifts from the meadow

Throughout history we have made allies of plants ...

Traditionally, it was the wise woman of the village to whom we went for help when a love-spell was wanted to secure a bond, when a child's fever needed quenching, when pain cried out to be soothed, or solace was sought for a soul in grief. According to archaeologists, this love affair between humans and plants goes back somewhere between 30,000 and 50,000 years – maybe more.

Take a walk in the country – no matter what country – any month of the year. Look around you. Even in the depth of winter, provided the ground is not covered with snow, you will find healing plants. Yesterday I went mountain biking in the South Island of New Zealand. It is early autumn here. The glorious summer plants have died back for the winter yet the fields, the verges of roads, the banks of the river we later floated down on inner tubes, were still riddled with healing plants. Stalks of mullein stood proudly by. They begged to be noticed and asked to be used. Huge hairy leaves of comfrey poked out from beneath the trees. These plants, which are not native to the Southern Hemisphere, had probably regenerated themselves from somebody's garden

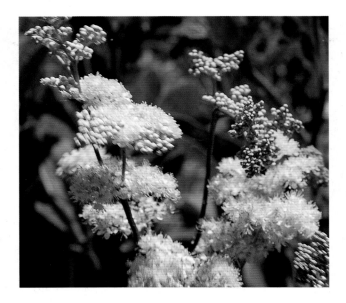

refuse dumped nearby. I found elderberries too, and plantain and yarrow.

All over the world, traditional herbal practices are centred on local plants. This makes a lot of sense. Local plants, like locally grown foods, are ideal for the people who live near them. But our lives have become global as have the herbs we use for health – from the rejuvenating Ayurvedic guggul to the Native American black cohosh, so useful in the treatment of female disorders. Likewise, the fascination with what plants can do for our health has become a world-wide phenomenon and not only when it comes to natural treatments either.

More than a quarter of drugs prescribed by doctors can be traced directly back beyond the abstract scientific laboratory in which they were formulated to the dense growth of the rainforest or the rich pickings of the meadow. One of the most popular drugs for high blood pressure, Reserpine, was originally derived from India's snake-root plant – a traditional remedy for snake bite. Even aspirin is the offspring of a European herbal remedy for pain and fever called Queen of the Meadow (*Filipendula ulmaria*), a 120 cm (4 ft) high perennial with gorgeous feathery, fragrant plumes that flowers in mid-summer. From quinine and codeine, to ephedrine and ipecac – all these medicines have their roots in herbs.

Nearly two-thirds of the planet's 260,000 flowering plants are native to the tropics. Multinational pharmaceutical companies from New York to Tokyo send their chemists into the dense vegetation of the rainforest. There they learn what they can from native healers in the search for plants unknown to the Western world. Back in their laboratories they work to isolate the so-called 'active ingredient' of a plant and see if it can be synthesized and turned into a patented drug. For it is only patented drugs, not natural remedies, that will earn their shareholders big dividends.

◄ queen of the meadow   ► evening primrose

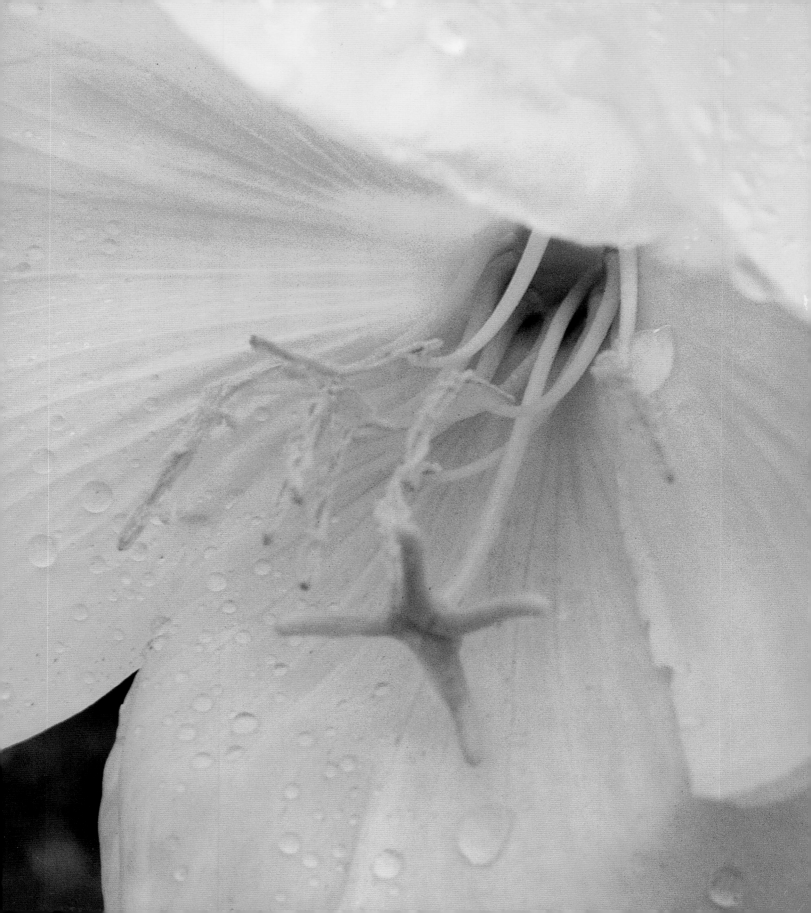

what is a herb?

The classic definition of a herb is a non-woody plant
that dies down to its roots each winter. Such a
description is far too limiting. It was probably made up
by nineteenth-century botanists who had never heard
of, let alone seen, the rainforest in which there is no
winter for anything to die back in. Neither would they
have ever heard of woody trees and shrubs such as
hawthorn, ginkgo and elder, which are some of the
best-selling herbs on the market these days. I define a
herb quite simply as a medicinal plant. It can come
from any climate and be a leaf, a bark, a flower or a
root. It can be home-grown or wild, a weed, a spice, a
plant that is used for its healing or culinary or
beautifying properties.

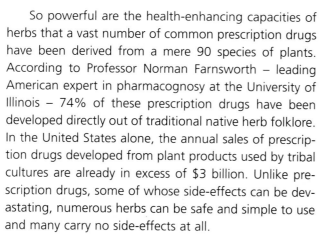

So powerful are the health-enhancing capacities of
herbs that a vast number of common prescription drugs
have been derived from a mere 90 species of plants.
According to Professor Norman Farnsworth – leading
American expert in pharmacognosy at the University of
Illinois – 74% of these prescription drugs have been
developed directly out of traditional native herb folklore.
In the United States alone, the annual sales of prescription drugs developed from plant products used by tribal
cultures are already in excess of $3 billion. Unlike pre-
scription drugs, some of whose side-effects can be devastating, numerous herbs can be safe and simple to use
and many carry no side-effects at all.

Plants have taught us a lot, yet there are still so
many herbal secrets yet to be revealed. At the turn of
the millennium less than half of a percent of the flowering plants on the earth have been explored for their
healing potentials. Sadly, in the scramble to exploit the
knowledge of traditional healers and the plants they
work with, much real knowledge of using herbs for
healing is being lost together with the plants themselves. And so many of the drugs that have so far been
manufactured as a result of herb research carry dangerous, sometimes life-threatening side-effects in their
wake. It is a growing awareness of this that is leading us
back to learn from the plants themselves how they can
heighten energy, enhance our looks and improve the
quality of our lives. It is this information, which I have
gleaned over many years, that fills these pages.

With a few exceptions – like poppies and evening
primroses – herbs truly are not glitzy and glamorous.
Their flowers tend to be small and, unless you look at
them very close up, not very special. The full flown
beauty and power of their life-giving energy is hidden
deep within just waiting for someone with a little vision
to call it forth.

herb explosion

For a time, herbal treatments were replaced by single-molecule, drug-based medicine. Now they are back in force and developing fast. The European market in phytopharmaceuticals – herbal remedies – is worth US$7 billion. Rising rapidly each year, it already exceeds the growth of the drug-based pharmaceutical market. The sales volume for herbs in Europe is half that of the global total for plant-based remedies. Germany leads the way with 26% of the world's developing market for herbal preparations. France comes second. In many ways this is not surprising since, in the United States alone, adverse drug reactions officially kill more than 100,000 people each year and harm another 2.2 million – according to a report published in the prestigious *Journal of the American Medical Association*.

Not that all herbs are safe. All need to be used with caution. Yet experts in botanical medicine agree that, in general, herbs are far safer than most drugs. Much valuable modern research into the effectiveness and safety of herbs comes from Germany. Their organization Kommission E issues 'Therapeutic Monographs on Medicinal Products for Humans' and publishes them in the *German Federal Gazette* or *Bundesanzeiger*. Each monograph on a herbal remedy includes its constituents, indications for use, contraindications, side-effects, interactions with other foods, plants or drugs, methods for administration, dosages, and general properties of therapeutic value.

Herbs are not only here to stay. They have come out of the realm of folklore and hit the mainstream. If you are not using them yet you are missing out on all the wonderful things they have to offer – from energy and rejuvenation to first aid and freedom from aches and pains, not to mention beautiful skin and a sanctified space in which to live and work.

the whole is greater

The wise woman tradition of herbal use, which is closely connected with medical herbalism, has developed out of centuries of experiment and recorded observation. It relies on this long history of hands-on practice to determine what plants to use for what condition, how much, when and for whom. Herbalists, whether they be simple country people using local plants for healing or highly trained herbal doctors from the Western, Ayurvedic or Chinese traditions, share a universal ethic of respect for the plants they use, for the people they use them on and for the earth from which they come. Herbalists understand that a plant's health-enhancing properties derive not from one or two active ingredients but from a complex living synergy between dozens of its chemical and energetic characteristics – and on the complex ways in which this particular herb interacts with our own biological systems when we take it.

Modern scientific research on the other hand focuses on the task of identifying specific active ingredients and testing them on animals – something no traditional herbalist would ever agree was a useful measurement of a herb's actions. Well does the herbalist know the truth – recently illuminated by leading-edge physics and biology – that the whole is greater than the sum of its parts. You can analyse every chemical in an apple, for instance, but you cannot expect that if you put all of these chemicals together it will make an apple. Only nature can do that. Plants and humans have interacted for a million years or more, yet there are still great chasms in the knowledge of human biochemistry, the understanding of plant biochemistry, and understanding the ways the two interact. When working with herbs, the most important thing to become familiar with is the ways in which, over long-term use, plants have shown themselves to be helpful. This is the best way to gain access to the great wealth of herbal knowledge and to make it work for you in your own life.

healing truths

The way we have thought about health and healing for the past century – what the experts call our biomedical model – has come to the limits of its usefulness. Conventional medical practices now look at the body as a collection of structures – bones and blood, cells and tissues. Treatment consists largely of acting on these structures in a symptomatic way. For instance, doctors give one drug to lower blood pressure or cholesterol, another to get rid of headaches or to put you to sleep. Whether medically prescribed or over-the-counter products, many of them carry negative side-effects. And few are concerned with improving functions. They concentrate instead on treating symptoms. Little of twentieth-century illness medicine has concerned itself with 'healing', choosing instead to focus on 'managing' illness and suppressing symptoms.

Herbal medicine, like all of the great natural approaches down through history, looks at things differently. It insists that at any level of biological organization – from chromosomes in our DNA all the way up to our eyes and toes, stomach and liver – the body has a stunning capacity for self-diagnosis and self-treatment. So much so that it can often remove damaged structures and renew them with new ones all on its own. An awareness of the natural capacity of living organisms as complex as ours to regenerate themselves is at the very core of using natural foods, water, air, movement therapies and, of course, herbs.

Chinese medicine – in my opinion the greatest of all natural approaches to healing – is functional medicine. It did not develop along structural lines as Western twentieth-century medicine did, nor did Ayurvedic and Unani medicine from India, nature-cure or herbalism in the West. Chinese pharmacopoeia is the richest in the world. Chinese doctors value plants for their ability to strengthen the body's functioning, heighten its own defences and improve immunity. They use herbs, as we are now just beginning to in the West, to extend longevity, to increase resistance to illness, to heighten energy and to calm disturbed emotions.

The new medicine – real healing in the twenty-first century – is turning away from symptomatic treatment towards an understanding of how to make use of water, food, light and air, in ever more effective ways, not only for curing illness but for helping people expand their experience of positive health. Plant medicine – the new herbalism – lies right at the centre of this whole-person, whole-planet approach.

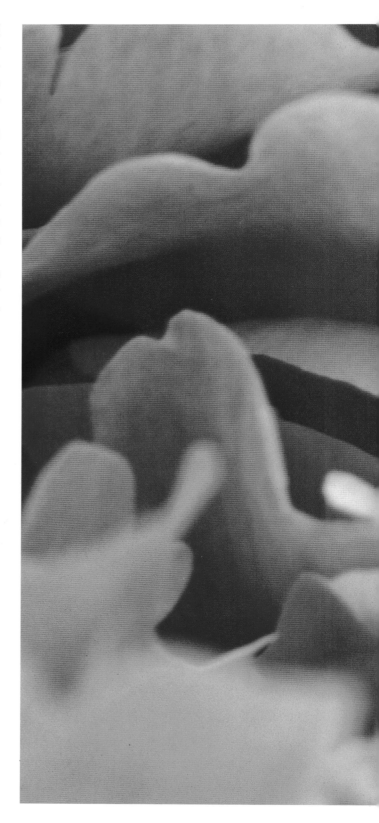

▶ peony root has been used for thousands of years in Chinese medicine for a wide range of aches and pains.

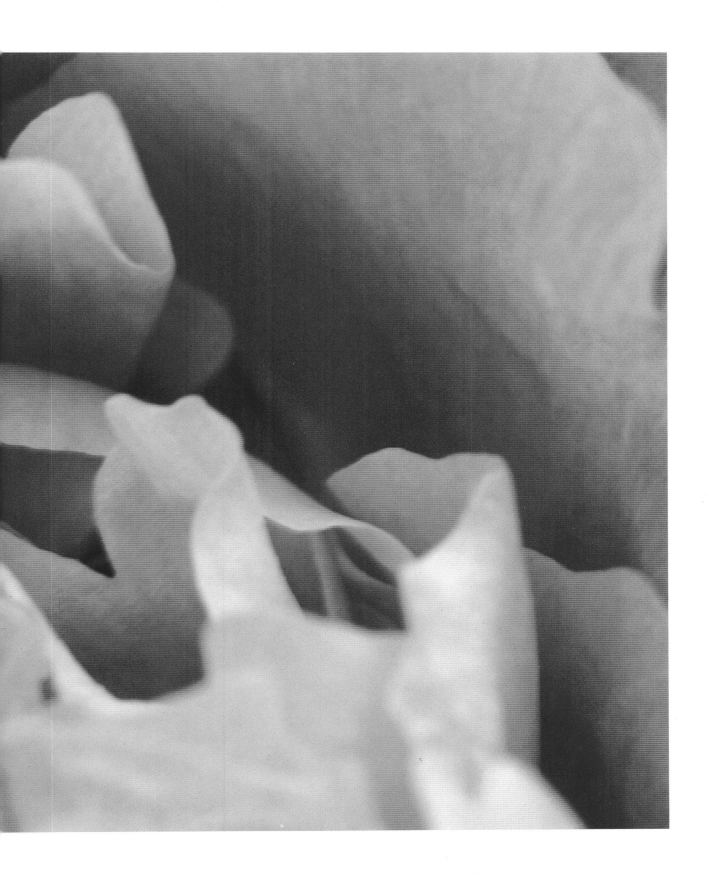

traditions old and new

According to both traditional practices and recent scientific experiments, the right plants can work wonders on the human body ...

aloe heals

The cool, slippery gel that oozes out of a leaf of the aloe cactus has been used for almost 3,000 years to treat burns and cuts and to undo the devastating effects of too much exposure to the sun. Recent studies show that phyto substances from the aloe actually penetrate damaged tissue, encouraging healing, increasing blood flow and easing inflammation and pain.

ginseng strengthens

The ancient Chinese said so and spent a fortune on this strange-looking man-root – they still do. Thousands of years ago ginseng was taken to extend life, to sharpen sexual functioning, to bring clarity to the brain and energy to the body. Russian and German scientists have carried out lengthy studies into the effects of ginseng on humans and animals and concluded that it does indeed sharpen the brain and shorten reaction time. It also improves concentration and helps protect you from damage caused by exposure to long-term stress.

garlic protects

The ancient Greeks, including Pliny in the first century AD, insisted that it banishes worms and coughs. By now there have been more than 2,500 studies that confirm its anti-microbial properties and its usefulness in warding off flu and colds, not to mention its ability to reduce blood pressure and cholesterol levels that are too high, and to help clear yeast infections.

comfrey knits

Its very name comes from the Latin *conferte* which means 'grow together'. In 400BC the Greek physician Dioscorides praised comfrey for its ability to stop heavy bleeding and clear bronchial infections. Science confirms that comfrey is rich in the healing compound allantoin, which enhances tissue growth and cell multiplication. That is why you will find it added to ointments and face creams.

ginger soothes

A core remedy in the Chinese pharmacopoeia for nausea and gentle cleansing, the deliciously hot ginger plant has been used for more than 1,500 years by wise women healers in Europe for tummy upsets. Several scientific studies confirm that it helps travel sickness. Some even show it helps morning sickness in pregnancy – in part because it has the ability to neutralize excess acid in the stomach.

feverfew banishes

Eccentric English herbalist Nicholas Culpeper sang the praises of this cheerful daisy-like plant with lacy leaves. It was, he claimed, 'effectual for all pains in the head'. Recent studies carried out in Britain confirm he knew what he was talking about. Feverfew can reduce both the frequency and the intensity of migraine.

tribal secrets

Tribal peoples knew the secrets of the living earth. Our ancestors were born and died in close proximity to the plants they used for food, for healing, for religious ceremonies. They were not only versed in each plant's physical properties, they intuitively sensed its unique sacred nature. They knew the beauty of each herb the way you know a child or a lover – its fragrance, its feel, its personality, and its touch. They were sensitive to when and how to gather a plant. And, because these men and women were also highly practical – believing to be true only what they experienced – our ancestors also knew

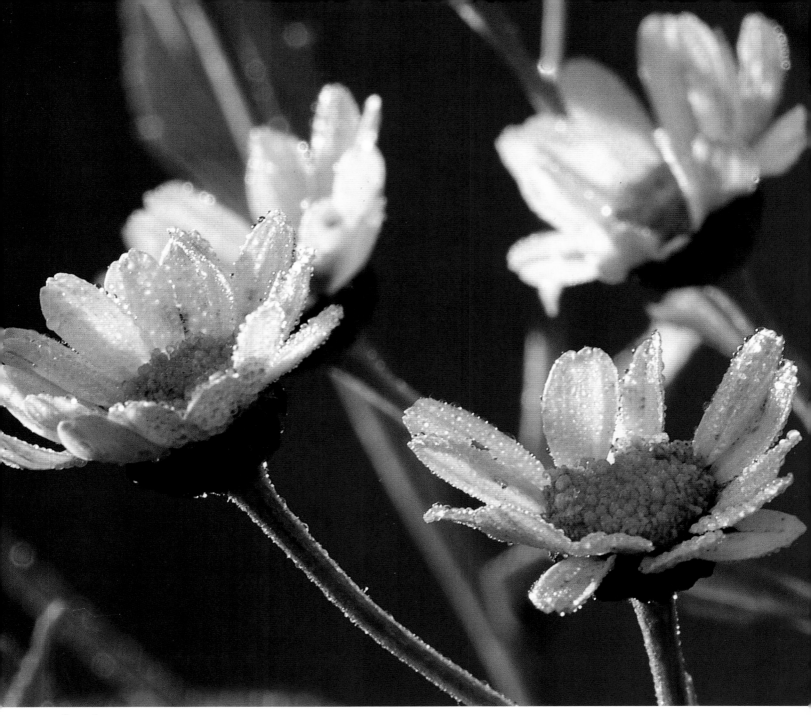

▲ feverfew

just how to call on the magic of a herb or flower, root or seed to whatever end they wished to apply it.

Modern urban life has robbed us of the wilderness in which we once lived out our love affair with plants, and ripped away much of the knowledge of herbs that was once passed on from generation to generation. It has also undermined our confidence in our ability to interact with plants and to form personal alliances with them that make great healing, beauty and joy possible. Rediscovering your connection with herbs not only helps strengthen your body and heightens your energy, it also makes you richer in spirit.

entering the sacred

The sacred is everywhere if only we have eyes to see it. From every rock and every stream it pours forth ...

Perceiving the sacredness of a plant or herb is a consciousness-expanding experience of incredible beauty. It encompasses our five senses yet takes us beyond them too, into the realms of intuition and instinct, which our left brain-orientated education tends to burn out of us.

In tribal cultures, people live with an awareness of the spiritual nature of the world around them. To them the earth is sacred, so is an animal, the changes of the seasons, the sun and the rain, the birth of a child, or the death of an elder. They relate to each of these things with expanded awareness – they are able not only to see the surface but also to penetrate deep into their subtle nature. They know divine energy that informs all life. They seek therefore to form highly personal relationships with the plants they eat, with the herbs they heal with, and the grasses they build their homes with. They look closely at them, smell them, touch them, penetrate the nature of their energies without ever stopping to think about it. As a result, they come to know which herbs are to be used to ease an aching back or heal a wound, to help a barren woman become fertile and put a crying child to sleep. Because the plants tell them.

Our modern world feels profoundly uneasy before such experiences. Yet anyone who has grown herbs, healed with them and worked with them, knows full well that each plant has a unique and deeply mysterious nature. When you feel your way towards a herb's sacred spirit, a magic takes place whereby you come to know its true nature, how it wants to be used, how you can best care for it and how best it can care for you. That is what entering into a sacred relationship with a plant is all about.

Every species of herb has a unique spirit. When we are able to tune into that our lives become infinitely richer. It is not hard to do. They also give us medicines and the air that we breathe.

the art of listening

It is not hard to learn to listen to a plant. All it requires is a little time and quiet. Sit before a herb or flower that attracts you. Reach out and touch its leaves and stems, its flowers and fruit. Look with soft eyes at it. Then close your eyes and imagine that you are this herb or plant. See what it feels like. Sense your roots going deep into the earth and your stems and branches reaching towards the light. If the plant before you were talking to you what would it want to tell you? If you wish, ask the plant if you can pick one of its leaves or flowers and then wait a moment and receive its reply intuitively. Thank the plant and return to ordinary consciousness. Van Gogh once said that it is looking at things for a long time that ripens you and gives you a deeper understanding. Try doing this with herbs. You may be surprised by how much you learn from them.

▶ Take a walk through a forest of sage. It can change your life. This common plant comes in many forms from red sage (*Salvia officinalis*), which as a gargle banishes sore throats, to desert sage (*Artemesia tridentata*), right. Each and every plant that bears the name sage has one thing in common: the power to cleanse negative influences at the very deepest levels – be they microbes in infections or energy fields in rooms. Burn desert sage and its aromatic properties smudge away whatever does not belong there on an energetic level and sanctifies the space.

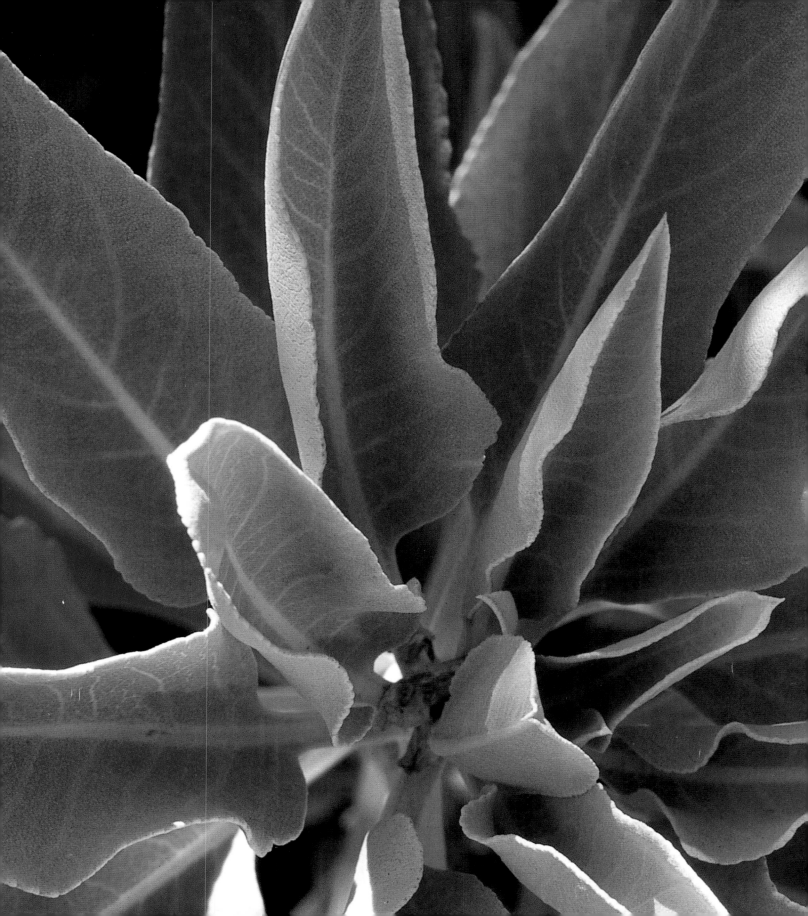

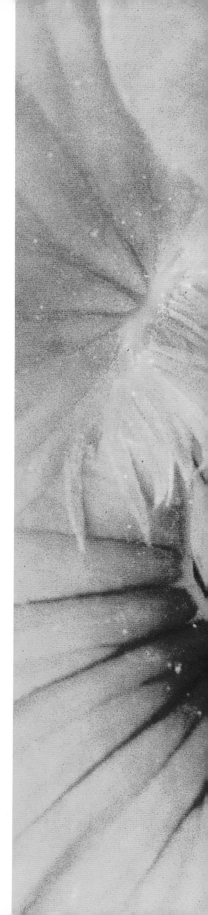

secrets of plant power

Herbs are enormously hardy. Like street
kids who grow up in tough surroundings,
these plants are survivors ...

Most have had to withstand harsh weather and little nourishment from the soil. This has helped clear out the weaklings and make their genetic strains stronger. This has also led them to develop an array of potent phytochemicals that are divided into groups such as alkaloids, flavonoids, saponins, tannins and phytosterols and they help describe the way a herb acts upon the body.

Knowing a little of phytochemistry only enriches your sense of wonder and respect for these living marvels of nature. What you need to remember is that it is not just the principal active ingredients that are important, it is the way all the elements of a plant can work with lesser active constituents to produce a life-enhancing synergy that makes herbs work for us (see chart on pages 26-27). Much research has been carried out into plant chemistry in an attempt to identify the most active ingredients.

These plant chemicals, which play a beneficial role in the developing herb, also bring us health when we use them. Take bitters, for instance. You find them in herbs like dandelion, mugwort, gentian, horehound, burdock and in yellow dock. Botanists believe bitter elements probably help protect the plant from being eaten in the wild. And they are wonderful for enhancing digestion. They help heal the lining of the gut, improve the way our digestive enzymes, juices and hormones work, and stimulate the flow of bile. Bitter herbs seem to validate that old saying that the worse something tastes, the better it is for you.

mind benders

Alkaloids – plant chemicals that botanists believe help regulate plant growth as well as discouraging predators – can have powerful effects on our mind when we use them. Coffee is full of them. So are opium, black tea, cocoa and tobacco. Many immune-enhancing plants such as echinacea and goldenseal, so useful in protecting from illness and clearing infection, are also rich in alkaloid compounds. Meanwhile, gums and resins like myrrh, pine, and the Ayurvedic remedy guggul, are taken from branches and woods and seem to carry the life blood of a tree or shrub. They transport nutrients to wherever the plant needs them. And some of these, such as guggul, can be useful in enhancing our own circulation and lowering cholesterol.

get into colour

The brilliant colours of flowers, stems, leaves and fruits are not just beautiful to look at. They are also rich in flavonoids – the phytochemicals responsible for vivid yellows

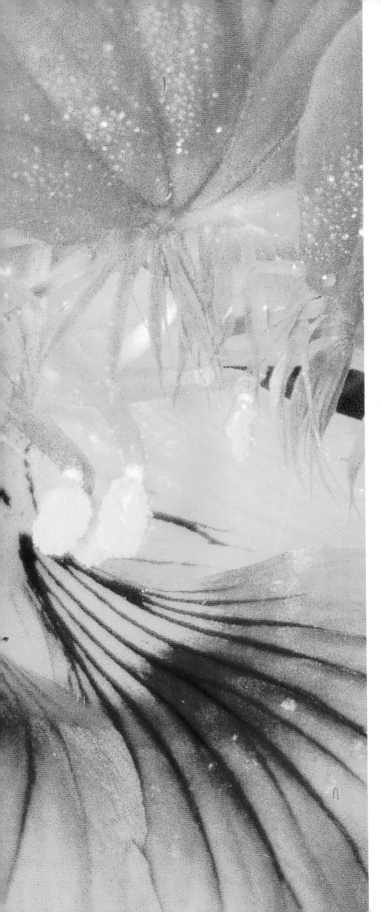

and oranges and reds that attract bees and other insects for pollination. These glorious living hues probably also attract animals. Then beasts who eat the plants unwittingly act as carriers for their seeds.

To the human body, flavonoids offer great anti-ageing health benefits. Many are powerful antioxidants against free-radical damage – even more powerful than the well-recognized vitamins A, C, E and the minerals selenium and zinc. They help protect us from degeneration, they strengthen our blood vessels and the collagen in our skin, they guard our cells from oxidation destruction, they calm inflammation and help keep the body free of water retention. Some flavonoids even help clear muscle spasm. The anthraquinones, found in the roots and leaves of herbs like yellow dock, protect plants from fungal and bacterial destruction. For us, plants rich in these yellow phytochemicals can help stimulate bile production, boost a sluggish liver and improve digestion.

sustaining saponins

The saponins that you find in roots and leaves lather like soap. Some are useful expectorants for coughs. Others help us regulate hormones or counteract stress. The essential oils of herbs, found in leaves and flowers, fruits and barks, help plants like mint, bergamot, lavender and ginger attract pollination thanks to their signature fragrances. Thanks to their antimicrobial actions, their essential oils also protect them from disease .

In our lives some essential oils make it possible for us to create beautiful perfumes and incense. Some have antiseptic actions, others improve digestion, stimulate circulation, improve the look and texture of skin and do a hundred other good deeds. It is fascinating to become familiar with the actions of phytochemicals. The more you learn about them the more you realize just how all-encompassing herbal healing can be.

◄ nasturtium and, overleaf, peppers and red cabbage. The chemicals that bring plants their colour are themselves phytonutrients.

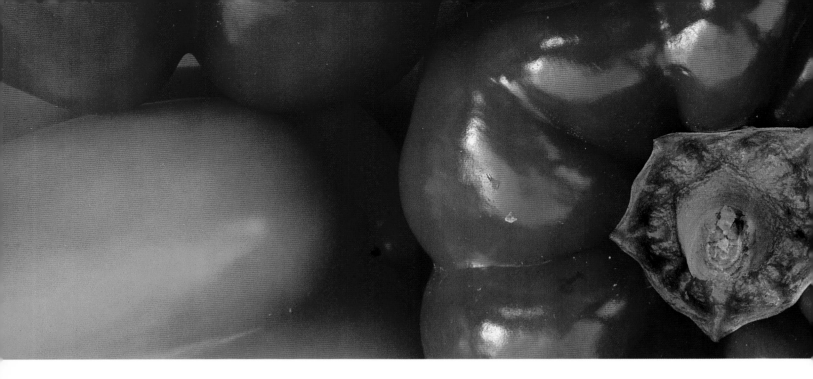

holistic phytochemistry and synergy

Alkaloids

◆ Alkaloids contain nitrogen, which produces alkaline reactions in the body. They are extremely potent. A few can even be deadly. Alkaloids extracted from plants include morphine and heroin from the opium poppy, atropine from deadly nightshade, caffeine from coffee, scopolomine from hellebore and mescaline from the peyote cactus. When alkaloids are present in herbs in small amounts (such as in comfrey) they act as a catalyst to the action of other constituents. In recent years, comfrey has been unfairly discredited. The herb itself will cause no damage. Comfrey root, on the other hand, is not available for human or animal consumption, as prolonged consumption has been deemed unwise.

Flavonoids

◆ Flavonoids are common substances which give an orange or yellow colour and a bitter-sweet taste to a plant. They have a wide range of effects on the body – diuretic, antispasmodic, heart stimulant. Some can lower blood pressure by strengthening the circulatory system. Flavonoids are heavy-duty anti-agers. You will find them in plants rich in vitamin C. Their presence improves the absorption of the vitamin in the body and enhances the look of skin.

Glycosides

◆ Glycosides produce sugars and therefore energy. They have a tonic and restorative effect on the body, and are often laxative and purgative as well. They include a group called the 'cardiac glycosides' which support and stabilize the heart while increasing its efficiency. Digitalis is a famous cardiac glycoside, although most herbalists today prefer to use the more gentle lily of the valley. Anthraquinones are another well-known group of glycosides. Bitter to taste and yellow in colour with a laxative effect, they have an ability to clear pathogens from the gut.

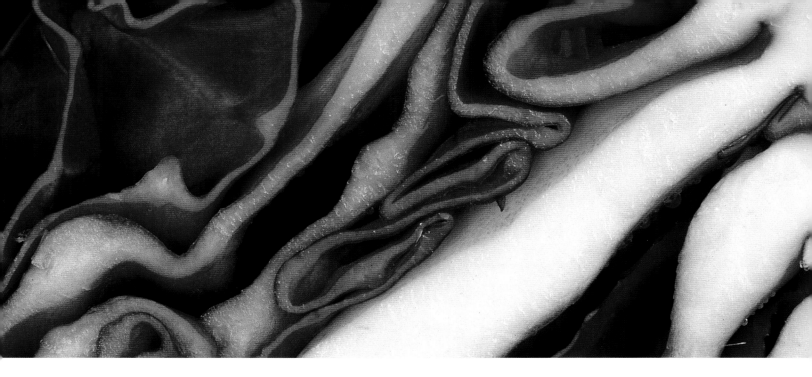

Phyto-steroids	◆ Phyto-steroids act like human hormones in the body even though they are not identical to them. They include oestrogen, testosterone, cortisol and cholesterol-like hormones. Although cholesterol has had a bad press recently it is worth remembering that the body needs cholesterol to produce many of its hormones. Cholesterol from plants tends to remain in the blood rather than be deposited on artery walls as it is accompanied by those substances (such as lecithin and choline) which help keep it in circulation where it belongs.
Saponins	◆ Saponins are sweet-tasting substances that form a lather when mixed with water and can emulsify oils. They aid the uptake of certain minerals and trace elements and can have diuretic and expectorant effects. Steroidal saponins are similar in structure to human hormones (see phyto-steroids). Most saponins are anti-inflammatory.
Tannins	◆ Tannins are sour-tasting astringent substances that cause tissues to contract. Tannins are able to bind a protein found in the skin and mucous membranes, albumin, so that they form a tight layer and protect from infection and reduce inflammation. They have been used throughout human history to tan the hides of animals as well.
Volatile or essential oils	◆ The most fascinating of all herbal constituents, volatile oils are often found in highly scented herbs frequently used in cooking. Although each of these complex hydrocarbons is made up of different chemical compounds – as many as 50 in some cases – they have common actions. Volatile oils are antiseptic and antibiotic. They stimulate the production of white cells and so aid the immune system. They also aid digestion and have an action on the central nervous system that is either calming or stimulating.

buying herbs

There is an endless parade of different ways you can use herbs ...

In health food stores, pharmacies and mail order catalogues – these days even in many supermarkets – you will find a confusing array of capsules, pills, tablets, extracts, tinctures and 'whole herbs' or 'bulk herbs', none of which seem to relate to the 'infusion' you have decided that you would like to take. And what about the herbs you have growing in your garden? Here is a rough guide to finding your way through the confusion.

discover your options

bulk dried or whole herbs

What you are buying is a bag or box of a specific weight of dried herb, either in its whole form, crushed, or powdered. This is the best way to purchase herbs if you want to make teas (infusions), decoctions, or your own capsules, or if you want to use them in potpourris and sachets. It is also the cheapest way to buy dried herbs.

tinctures

A tincture uses alcohol diluted in water to draw out the plant's chemical constituents, which dissolve in alcohol, and then to preserve them. You can buy tinctures by the bottle. They are pretty potent. Take roughly ½ to 1 teaspoon of an average strength tincture in a little water at a time. Tinctures are best bought from a reputable supplier. You can make them yourself but the process is less accurate than when they are professionally produced. I buy many herbs in tincture form as this is convenient.

You will sometimes find a figure such as 1:4 written on a bottle of tincture. This gives you the ratio of the weight of the herb (in this instance, 1 part of herb) to alcohol/water mix (in this case, 4 parts). A herbalist may suggest you take a specific ratio, in which case your supplier can advise, but for general usage you shouldn't need to know the ratio.

fluid extracts

Extracts are sometimes confused with tinctures, yet they are far more concentrated. They aim to contain all the active chemicals of the plant, not only those that will dissolve in alcohol. Extraction processes vary from pressure rolling and heat treatment to vacuum extraction. They are best left to the experts. Extracts have a limited shelf life too and they should be kept in the fridge. Herbalists often prescribe extracts during an illness rather than using them for prevention. Extracts are also useful to add to a cream or salve for external use: mix 1 part extract into 3 parts base. They are pretty strong in their action.

solid extracts

A solid extract is a fluid extract that has had all of the solvent removed. The solid that is left is then dried and powdered and made into tablets or put into capsules. In solid extracts the measurement 4:1 would mean that 4 parts of the whole herb were used to make 1 part of solid extract. The more parts whole herb that are used to make one part of solid extract, the stronger it will be – 10:1 is therefore twice as strong as 5:1.

tablets, pills and capsules

Tablets, pills and capsules are available in health food stores and chemists, often more readily than the loose dried herbs themselves. Tablets, pills and capsules usually contain the whole herb, not just the constituents extracted in a tincture or infusion. Therefore in taking them you are making use of the synergy in action between all the constituents of each plant. Choose those from a reputable manufacturer/supplier.

Tablets are made from dried plant material – leaves, roots, bark and/or flowers – mixed with a base, sometimes lactose, both to help you hold them in your hand to take them and to aid absorption in the stomach.

Pills are tablets with a coating. If the plant is sticky, smelly, tastes dreadful – or all three – it is more likely to come in pill form than tablet as the protein or sugar coating disguises less pleasant aspects of the plant.

Capsules, made of gelatine or a vegetarian equivalent, are filled with dried herbs – even the stickier, smellier ones. They need to be stored in a cool, dry place. You can buy gelatine capsules from a chemist and fill them yourself either with herbs you have dried or with dried herbs you have bought in bulk. The standard 00 size capsule holds about ½ gram (500 mg) of herb. Make sure the herb is ground into as fine a powder as possible before filling so that it can be easily absorbed by the body.

buy the best

First find yourself a reputable supplier. I have listed a few under Resources, but you may have a good local supplier who is even better. Personally, I am wary of buying herbs in health food stores or pharmacies unless they are from a manufacturer or supplier I know. With a supplier you trust and with whom you can discuss your needs you can be sure you are getting a good potency and that the herbs have not been sitting in a cupboard somewhere for years.

It is up to us to make sure that the herbs we choose – like everything else we buy – are the very best quality. This is especially important now since the growth in herbal products in recent years has been so fast that everybody wants to get in on the act. As a result, on shop shelves you will find good guy herbs – those skilfully prepared tinctures, extracts and encapsulated herbs that are clean, fresh and brimming with life-enhancing properties – next to very poor quality products. The bad guy herbs include plants that have been irradiated, 'cut' with inert fillers to make them go further, or contaminated by herbicides and pesticides. Herbs that are too old will have lost their potency.

Look for well-tested products whose brand names have been around for a long time. Although this is by no means a guarantee of excellence, herbal suppliers have their reputation to consider and those with a good name have usually earned it. It can sometimes be a good plan to go for single herb products, as complex mixtures from mediocre suppliers often contain inadequate doses of each plant. You can also write direct to any herb supplier whose products you want to check out and ask a few pointed questions.

standardization

Pick up a bottle of herbs and you may find a word written on it which was never used a decade ago: standardized. St John's wort, for instance, is often standardized – which means guaranteed to contain at least 0.3% hypericin. Milk thistle is standardized to 70% silymarin, Ginkgo biloba is standardized to 24% flavone glycosides and 6% terpene lactones.

The practice of standardizing originated in Germany and the United States in an attempt to guarantee that a customer buying the herb will get a specific quantity of a plant's biologically active compounds – that which is believed to carry the plant's therapeutic effects. There is some sense in this since levels of a plant's most active ingredients can vary widely depending on how it has been grown and where, how it was gathered, processed – even the time of day at which it was harvested. It is particularly sensible when – as some herbalists do – you are using a plant not for its holistic healing power but as a source of a particular chemical which is being given much as a conventional doctor might prescribe a drug.

questions to ask

◆ How was the plant processed?
◆ Have you verification that it was not sprayed with chemicals in the growing process?
◆ What quality control procedures does the company have in place?
◆ Do you have a certificate of authenticity of the genus and species of the plant used?
◆ What part of the plant was used?
◆ What solvents have been used in preparing a tincture?
◆ Was the plant irradiated?

triple confusion

There are three ways of standardizing herbal products for consistent levels of at least some of their ingredients:

◆ Extract the principal active compound by dissolving the whole herb in alcohol or some other solvent such as hexane to create a tincture.

◆ Blend various batches of herbal extracts – including tinctures – in an attempt to get a product with a specified level of active ingredient.

◆ Add an extra 'active ingredient' to the product.

You never know which approach has been used when you see 'standardized' on the label for the whole area of standardization is not defined by any government body nor is the process controlled. It is carried out in whichever of these ways a supplier decides to carry it out.

There are some herbs which I believe can benefit from standardization. In the case of these plants standardization gives you the chance to have a good idea of what you are buying since there are now many products on the market containing these particular herbs, some of which will be very poor quality. The herbs you might consider buying in standardized form are these: calendula, camomile, echinacea, evening primrose, ginseng, ginkgo, hawthorn, kava kava, liquorice, milk thistle, olive leaf extract and tea tree.

go the whole way

In general, however, I prefer to use either the whole herb or products made from whole herbs. I look for those made from plants that have been grown in healthy soils – preferably organic – and have been properly harvested and skilfully processed with great respect for the natural healing powers they contain and a desire to bring them to market as much as possible intact. I prefer whole herbs for two reasons. First, when you mess about with a plant, adding this and taking that away, readjusting chemical ingredients, you disrupt a plant's natural healing synergy and may lose some of its sacred power in the process.

Second, there is an amusing arrogance in the assumption that we are sure what the so-called 'active ingredient' is in a particular plant. You could be buying a herb in which a particular ingredient has been standardized only to find out a year or two later that scientists have discovered that this ingredient is actually not the most active ingredient as had been believed. Or you might discover that to work its best, this so-called active ingredient needs to be in the presence of yet another active ingredient, which has been ignored in the standardization process. This happened recently in the case of St John's wort when researchers discovered that the plant chemical they were standardizing for may not at all be the most active.

After all is said and done, I am more likely to purchase a tincture of echinacea or camomile which has not been standardized than one which has. So, although I respect the process of standardization and sometimes use standardized herbs myself, I guess I respect the wisdom of nature even more.

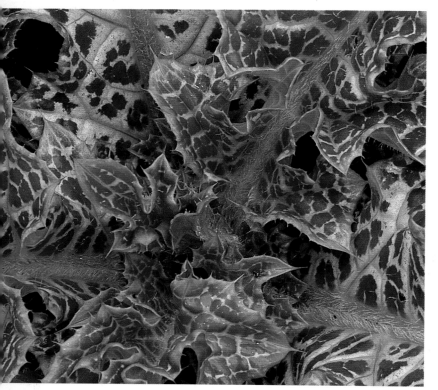

▲ milk thistle   ▶ marigold

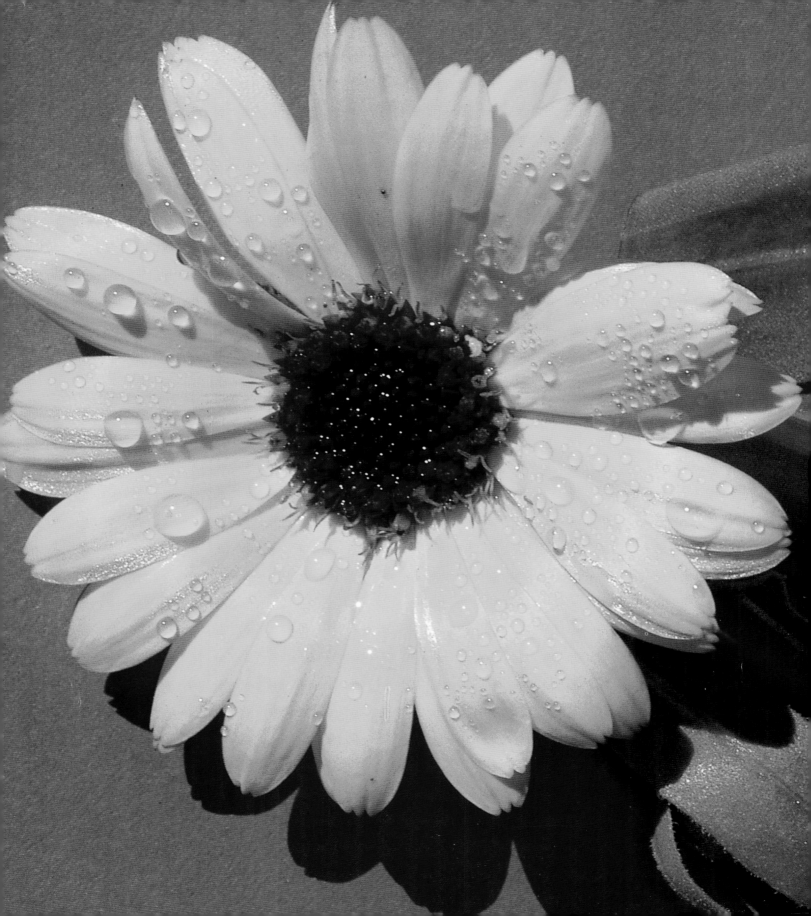

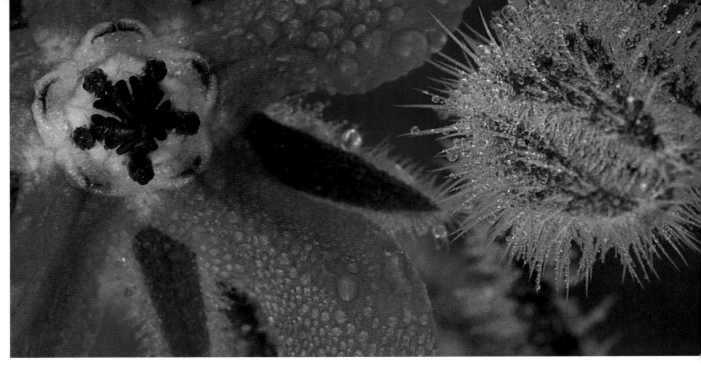

▲ borage

DIY herbs

There are many, many books devoted to the pleasure and skill of growing herbs in your own garden, so I won't go into detail here. Suffice it to say that the most common ones – plants such as the mints, borage and comfrey – are not hard to grow so long as you use common sense and don't try growing Mediterranean herbs in clay soil where a cold north wind blows. Once you've grown them, don't forget to harvest them.

fresh is best

Don't be afraid to cut bits off your herbs. They love it. It will only help them grow stronger and bushier. So make use of them. It's silly to use last year's dried herbs when you have fresh ones in abundance outside. You can make fresh teas and use them every day in cooking and salads. A note of caution, however. Before you go tearing around the hedgerows remember that it is against the law to pick most wild flowers. Growing them in your own garden and picking them is fine. You can get a good selection of herbs and wild flower seeds in your local garden centre and from specialist growers. Also, if you find something growing wild in your garden that you think is a herb, check in at least two good books first and preferably ask someone who knows about herbs to identify it. It can be easy to confuse some common species.

dry your herbs

Drying plants is easy and lots of fun too. Here are a few general rules-of-thumb. You will find you learn quickly as you go along. Gather your flowers immediately after they open but only after any dew or rain has dried from them. Gather leaves just before the flower fades – again when dew or rain has dried. If you want the whole plant, pick it when the flowers are open. If you want stalks, seeds or barks, gather them in the autumn.

Dry your plants in small bunches hanging upside down out of the sun to preserve their aromatic oils. Most herbs will dry in just a couple of weeks, others can take anything up to a year. You can also dry leaves and flowers by spreading them out in a single layer on paper or a screen so that air can circulate around them. This is the best way of drying roots, but you will need to slice the larger ones. Once you have dried them completely store the plants in glass jars. Brown glass is the best as it reduces the amount of light getting to the herbs. Make sure the plants are fully dry or they will rot. And be careful to label your jars properly, including a date.

using herbs

A beginner's guide to
herbal remedies for ease of
reference ...

infusions

A herbal infusion is nothing more than a herb tea. It is usually made from the fresh or dried 'soft' parts of the plant – leaves, stems and flowers – to bring out the vitamins and volatile oils. Teas are sometimes also made from seeds or roots. A general rule is to put 1-2 teaspoons of dried herb in a cup or tea pot and pour a cup of just boiled water over them. You will need to use more of the fresh herb – 2 to 3 times the dried quantity. Leave your tea to stand (steep) for 5 to 20 minutes, depending on the herb. Strain and drink. Whatever your good intentions, you won't drink a herb tea that tastes nasty. Adding pleasant-tasting herbs to your brew such as mint, fennel, lavender and liquorice will help. Infusions keep if refrigerated, but only for a day or two.

decoctions

A decoction mostly uses the woody parts of the plant – bark, seeds, roots and nuts – to get at the mineral salts and bitter principles and instead of being steeped the plants are simmered. You drink it like a tea. First, break open seeds and nuts and crush the roots and barks (a pestle and mortar are good for this), then bring them to the boil in a pan of water. Pouring boiling water over them isn't enough to extract their goodness. You will need to use slightly more water in a decoction to allow for some of the water boiling away. Cover the pan and simmer your herbs for 10 minutes before straining.

tinctures

Tinctures take a little more time but they are not hard to make. Tinctures will keep for a year or two. You use them in small quantities. You can use brandy, vodka or rum as your solvent. They already have water mixed with the alcohol. Use 100 g (4 oz) of dried herb or 225 g (8 oz) of fresh plant to 600 ml (1 pint) of your chosen alcohol. Put your herbs into a glass jar with a well-fitting lid and pour the alcohol over them. Close the lid tightly and keep the jar in a warm place for two weeks, giving it a good shake twice a day.

Strain your mixture through muslin until you have just a herb mash left in your cloth. Squeeze the mash out well and then pour the liquid into a clean – preferably sterilized – bottle with a lid and keep it refrigerated.

You don't have to refrigerate tinctures unless you live in a very hot climate but I prefer to store them this way since it keeps them fresh even longer and preserves the plant activity. Tinctures will last longer in brown glass bottles, which protect them from the light.

syrups

Syrups are good for coughs and colds, and for people who can't take the taste of herbs in the raw. But store them in the refrigerator in bottles with corks as they can ferment and have been known to explode. The basic formula for a syrup is 225 g (8 oz) of honey to which you add 250 ml (8 fl oz) of infusion or 125 ml (4 fl oz) of tincture mixed with 125 ml (4 fl oz) of water. You may have to warm the honey first to make sure the herb infusion or tincture can be thoroughly mixed in. Because honey is naturally antibacterial it makes much better syrups than sugar, which is the old-fashioned way of making them. Use 1-3 teaspoons of syrup several times a day when you need it.

ointments

A quick and simple way to make an ointment is to mix your herb with Vaseline. You do this by cooking the herb in the Vaseline in a double-boiler. Melt the Vaseline and keep it on a low heat. Add 2 tablespoons of either dried or fresh herbs to 200 g (7 oz) of Vaseline. Cook for 10 minutes. Pour the mixture through muslin, squeeze out well and keep the liquid in a sealed container.

I am not that keen on using petroleum-based products. So, if like me you prefer another means a slightly more complex recipe, using calendula and comfrey, is given below. Ointments use herbs that are good for skin healing. They are great for first aid.

You can buy arnica, comfrey and calendula ointments from health food shops and reputable herbal suppliers (see Resources). I like to mix comfrey and calendula in the same ointment so I prefer to make my own. I tend to make double quantities of the base then split it in two. That gives me the chance to make one ointment with arnica and the other with calendula and comfrey. You can make a comfrey ointment and then a calendula ointment if you prefer to apply them separately.

st john's wort oil

You can buy this bright red oil from good herbal suppliers (see Resources). But it is so simple to make for yourself.

compresses/fomentations

They may sound like they have come out of a medieval tract on hell, but compresses and fomentations are fast and effective tools for healing. Applied externally to speed the healing of injuries, they also ease inflammation, congestion and areas of pain. Compresses can be either hot or cold. Fomentations are generally hot.

hot compress or fomentation
You need a piece of clean cotton, gauze, or linen – a pillowcase slit open down its long sides and opened flat is ideal. Soak the cloth in a hot infusion or decoction of the chosen herb. Wring it out, shake to cool it, fold it if necessary and put it directly on the skin over the affected area. Cover it with a towel to keep the heat in. Re-soak the cloth and re-apply when it cools down.

cold compress
Cold compresses use the same procedure but instead allow the decoction or infusion to cool. Putting it in the freezer or adding ice cubes is also a good idea.

poultices

A poultice is also an ancient but effective remedy. You apply it like a compress. They are famed for their ability to draw out toxins and to relieve congestion. Instead of soaking a cloth in either a decoction or infusion, in a poultice you use the whole plant – fresh or dried. Place

calendula and comfrey ointment

▶ *2 tbsp almond, apricot or grapeseed oil*
▶ *1 tsp beeswax*
▶ *2 tsp of tincture (2 tsp tincture of arnica, calendula or comfrey. For my calendula and comfrey ointment add 1 tsp of calendula and 1 tsp of comfrey tincture.)*

Put the oil and beeswax in a double boiler and allow the beeswax to dissolve into the oil, stirring well. Test by dropping a little on a plate and allowing to cool at room temperature. It should be soft enough to scoop from a jar. If it's too runny add a little more beeswax until you have a good consistency. Stir in your tincture. Allow it all to cool a little and then pour your mixture into jars. Seal it straight away and store your ointment in a cool, dark place. It should keep for up to a year.

st john's wort oil

▶ *St John's wort flowers*
▶ *olive oil*
▶ *cheesecloth or baby muslin*

Pick the flowers late in the summer, being careful not to stain your fingers with its distinctive red oil. Leave them to release some of their moisture overnight so they are well wilted. Chop them up and put them in a glass jar and cover with olive oil. Then add another 5 cm (2 in) of olive oil on top. Cover with cheesecloth or baby muslin for the oil will go mouldy if moisture is not allowed to escape. Put the jar in a warm, sunny place for three weeks (a greenhouse is a good place). Pick up the jar and swirl it all around gently each day. Strain your oil and bottle it. Store it in a cool, dark place.

bruised, fresh herbs (or a warm paste of dried herbs mixed with a little hot water) between two pieces of gauze and apply to the skin. Hold it in place with a thin bandage and keep warm with a hot-water bottle.

infused oils

You can make simple infused herb oils for use in cooking, to pour on salads, and to use as externally applied remedies such as St John's wort oil (see below opposite). To make an infused oil, pack a glass jar with your fresh herb and pour olive oil over it until the jar is almost full. Leave a little space at the top of the jar. Put a lid on the jar and leave in a warm place, preferably on a sunny windowsill, for two to three weeks. Give the jar a good shake daily. Strain the oil through muslin, squeezing out the leaves. Store in a brown glass jar in the refrigerator.

infused vinegars

The uses of herb vinegars are so many it is hard to list them all. You can make them with culinary herbs like basil, sage, garlic, thyme, or marjoram to use in your salad dressings. Alternatively, you can pour an infused vinegar made from your favourite perfumed herb into your bath to restore the skin's natural pH balance, which is naturally slightly acid. Or how about pouring a vinegar or two over your hair as a final rinse after shampooing. You can even take a dessertspoon of herb vinegar to cure hiccoughs.

medicinal wines

Medicinal, or tonic, wines are delicious and easy to make. The alcohol in the wine draws out the beneficial properties of any herb you soak in it, just like a tincture. But whereas you only take tinctures in small amounts, you can sip medicinal wines by the glassful. They are wonderfully restorative to the spirit.

You can make them with good quality red or white wine. Some herbs – roots such as ginseng or dang quai – suit red wine, whereas the delicate flowers of elder or camomile go well with white wine. Borage, rosemary and lemon balm go well with either.

If you use red wine you might like to add a little powdered ginger, a cinnamon stick or some grated nutmeg to make a rich, spicy tonic wine infused with the spirit of Christmas.

thyme herb vinegar

▶ *300 ml (½ pint) cider vinegar*
▶ *300 ml (½ pint) spring water*
▶ *2 tbsp fresh thyme*

Put the cider vinegar into a small glass jar with the spring water. Add the fresh herb, put the lid on the jar and leave it in a warm place – an airing cupboard is ideal. After ten days strain the vinegar and bottle it.

medicinal wine

▶ *large handful fresh herb such as borage, rosemary or lemon balm, or 100 g (4 oz) dried*
▶ *600 ml (1 pint) wine*

Crush the herbs slightly to release their essential oils and put them in a jar. Pour the wine over the herbs and seal the jar. Leave it in a cool place for one week if you have used flowers and leaves, two weeks if you have used tough roots like ginseng. Strain, and store the wine in a clean – preferably sterilized – bottle.

essential oils

Many herbs contain remarkable essential oils that can exert immediate effects on mind and body. NEVER take them internally, for even a very small amount of some of these essences can be poisonous. The best essential oils you can buy have been made using complex distillation processes to ensure the oils are as pure as possible. They can be said to contain the 'life force', or 'essence' of the plant. Essential oils are always used sparingly. A few drops will do the trick, any more can be overwhelming, even dangerous. You can add 3 or 4 drops to your bath (see page 63), put a few drops in an essential oil diffuser to fill your room with wonderful scents (see page 90), or make a delicious massage oil. Each oil has its own physical and psychological effects.

To make a simple massage oil use 1 drop of essential oil to each teaspoon of a pure fruit oil such as almond or apricot oil. A capsule of vitamin E squeezed into the oil when you mix it helps keep it fresh longer. You can make soothing massage oils with lavender, geranium or camomile.
Uplifting oils would be made from cinnamon, bergamot, patchouli or jasmine. Lavender or rosemary are good for mild aches and pains.

◄ bergamot

► wild garlic

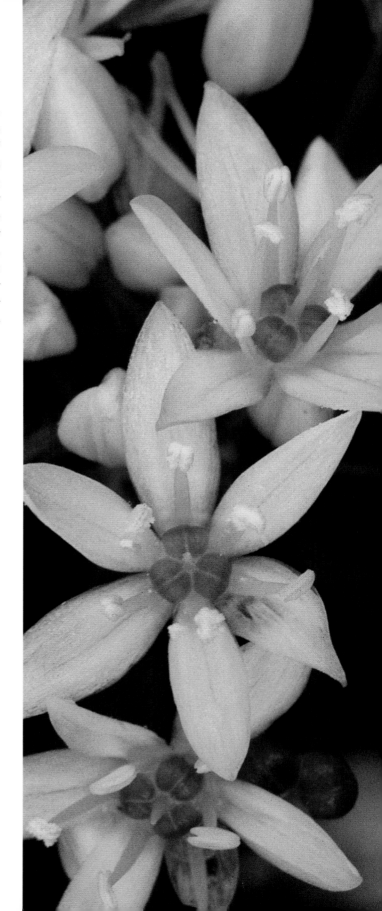

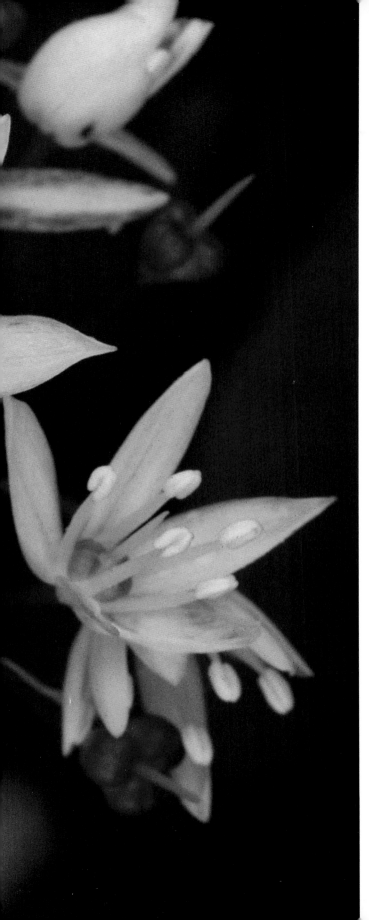

safe and sane

Don't become so
enthusiastic about herbs
that you go overboard ...

It is not wise to take lots of different plants all at the same time. You might start to think that since a small amount of something is good for you, taking two or three times that amount will be even better. It isn't. Here are a few guidelines to follow:

◆ Herbs occasionally interact with conventional drugs. Be sure to tell your doctor that you intend to try a herbal remedy.
◆ If you want to use herbs to treat a serious medical condition, find yourself a good medical herbalist to work with. Don't do it yourself.
◆ Take no more than recommended dosages of a herb or combination. If you notice any adverse reaction, stop right away.
◆ Use only the very best herbs, whether they be fresh, dried, teas, tinctures, extracts, or capsules.
◆ Give plants enough time to work. Many herbs, such as St John's wort and wild yam, are slow to build beneficial effects on the body. Look to six weeks for results.

go wild

The best way to use most herbs is to go into the wild and munch on them. I say this with very little tongue in cheek. Everywhere there are wild plants that offer health-enhancing benefits to people who can recognize them and know how to use them. I pick wild garlic in spring and put it in my salads knowing that not only will it make them more delicious, it will also help protect me and my family from minor illness thanks to its anti-microbial properties. I gather young, fresh nettles and bring them home to make tea. I reach for a handful of comfrey leaves, scrunch them up and press them against painful bruises and sprains.

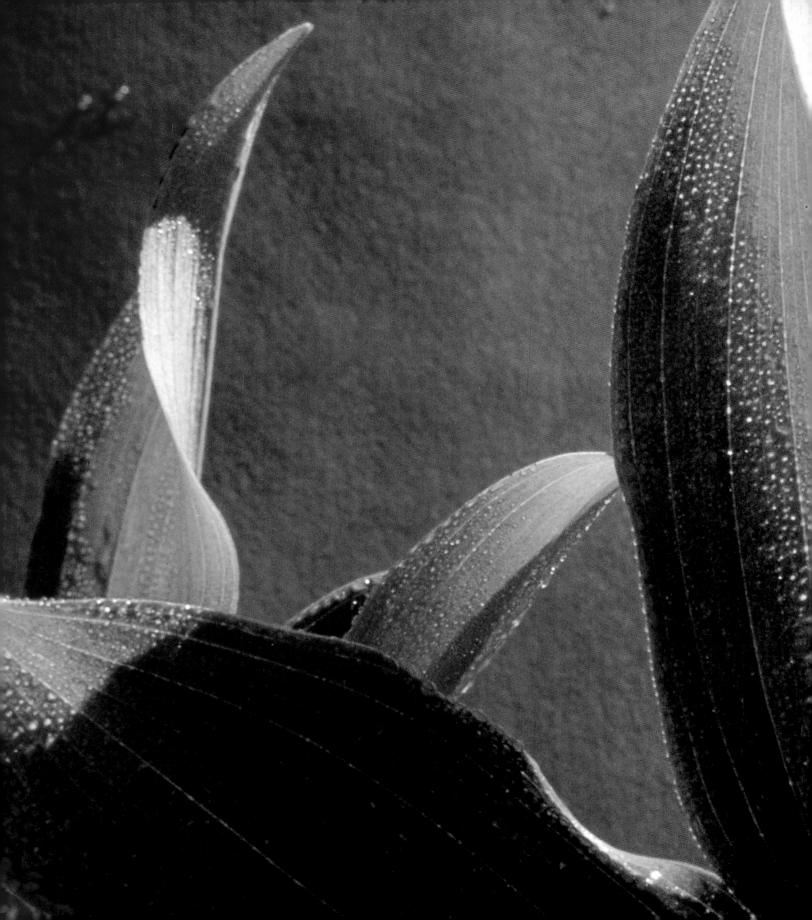

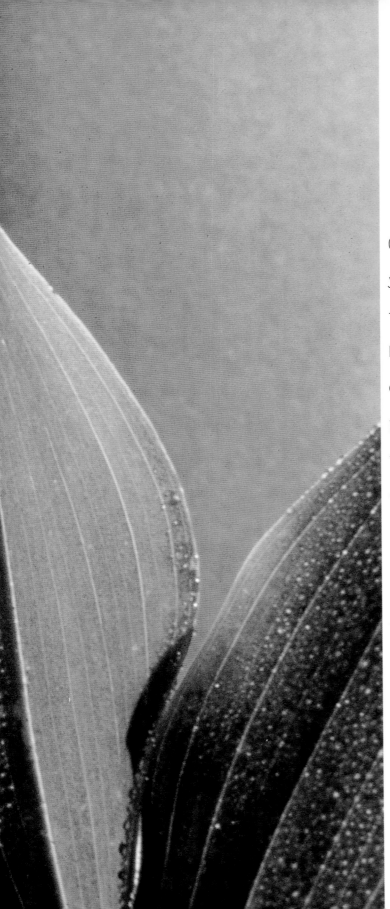

cleansing 2

Cleanse your body and it frees your spirit. This is an ancient truth known to every natural healer. The experience of detoxification is one of profound transformation leading towards a life of greater energy, clarity and joy. Deep cleansing is the beginning of healing, rejuvenation and regeneration. Let herbs be your catalyst. Like the sacred phoenix consumed by fire only to rise again, you will emerge in a dazzling new form.

◄ solomon's seal

leslie's herbal cleanse

Detox has become a buzzword at the millennium.
But don't be deceived into thinking that it is a
short-lived fad of dubious benefit ...

A programme to eliminate toxins from the body has been the foundation of natural medicine throughout history. There are numerous diets available to cleanse your body of stored wastes and clear toxicity. You can use them once or twice a year, whenever you feel you need them. But few make use of the most effective tools for detoxification: simple herbs.

clear it now

How do you know if you need a detox? However healthy your diet and however fit and active you are, it is difficult to avoid building up toxins in your system. We meet them in our food, our water, even in the air we breathe. A build-up of stored wastes puts a lot of strain on your liver, kidneys and intestines. It's a bit like carrying too many bags of shopping. The further you have to go with them, the worse the burden gets, the slower you go, and the more convinced you become that you don't need what's in the bags anyway. An overburdened body can produce all manner of problems as a direct result of toxicity – from weight gain, constipation, persistent coughs, itching, nausea, bloating, muscle or joint pains, poor sleep habits, digestive troubles, shortness of breath, irritability, low self-esteem, susceptibility to colds and flu, ageing skin or problem skin, chronic fatigue, even a sense of powerlessness. If you experience any of these symptoms, it could be time for a Herbal Cleanse.

The benefits of detoxifying are enormous. First, you can't build healthy new tissue without getting rid of old cells and their by-products. Second, helping your body throw off months and years of accumulated waste rejuvenates skin, pares off excess weight and strengthens your immune system. It can also put an end to digestive problems and aches and pains, increase your energy and

bring you clear eyes, bright spirits and shiny hair. If you have never used herbs to detox you are likely to be pleasantly surprised by how much easier and more thorough they make the whole process. Especially the fabulous trio: dandelion, cleavers and burdock.

The principal centres of elimination are the liver, the kidneys and the lymph system. Dandelion, burdock and cleavers work together to increase urine flow through the kidneys. Cleavers stimulates the kidney's processing of it. Where increased urine flow can sometimes result in a depletion of valuable minerals, dandelion and burdock combine to replenish any minerals lost. Meanwhile, cleavers exerts its influence on the lymphatics, so completing the threefold process that means efficient elimination can happen easily. Together, these three herbs pack quite a punch, yet their effects are balanced so they won't knock you off your feet.

The Herbal Cleanse lasts for just eight days. Unlike other detox programmes, thanks to the hard work put in by the herbs, the Herbal Cleanse does not demand you stick to a rigid diet. You can feast on fresh, wholesome and delicious foods that you choose for yourself. But you will need to cut out things like tea, coffee, alcohol and processed foods so you can let the herbs get on with removing toxins already in your system without you putting more in.

As stored wastes are eliminated from your body your skin will take on a new glow and translucence. Lines on your face will be softened and your eyes will become clear and bright. Your mind will become sharper so that thinking is easier. It is no accident that throughout history saints and philosophers have turned to abstinence – another way to cleanse the body and psyche – as a way of increasing spiritual awareness and improving mental clarity.

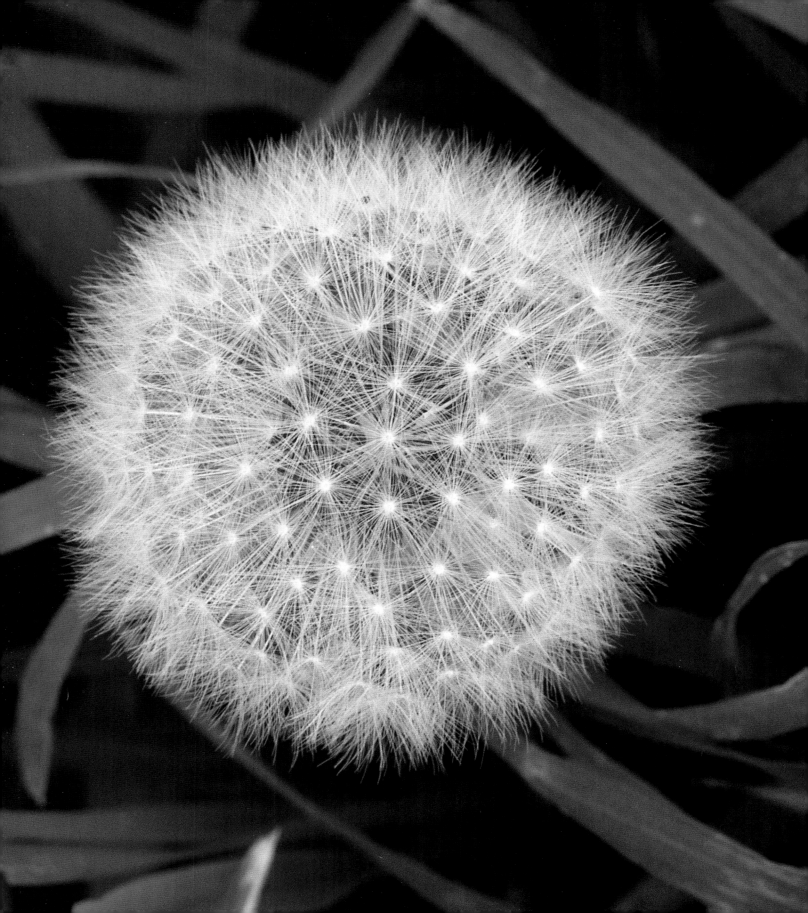

the dynamic three

Dandelion, burdock and cleavers ...

Before you begin your cleanse, prepare your daily herbal formula. You can take it either as an extract, a tincture in water, or in capsules, it's up to you. If you choose to take capsules you will need only 42 of each (see chart below), size 0, for the programme. If you buy more than this, they will keep fresh in the refrigerator or freezer for the next time. If you prefer to take your formula as a tincture, as I do, you will need roughly 100 millilitres each of dandelion, burdock and cleavers. Some herbal suppliers sell their tinctures in larger quantities than this but they too will keep well in the refrigerator for later use (see Resources).

For a really easy way to take your tinctures measure out enough of each for the week and mix them together. Store your mixture in a dark glass bottle and measure out 3 teaspoons into water at a time. Extracts are another easy way to take your daily herbal formula and as they are stronger than tinctures you will need to take less of them – only 20 drops of each fluid extract (roughly ⅓ of a teaspoon) at a time. Keep them in the refrigerator so they maintain their effect.

You can, if you feel confident enough to do so, pick, dry and powder your own herbs. But be very, very sure that you have correctly identified the plants as burdock in particular can be confused with other, similar looking wild plants

strong as a lion

As the brilliant yellow lion's mane of the familiar dandelion (*Taraxacum officinale*) pushes its way arrogantly through your lawn, you may curse its presence and despair at the length and strength of its roots, but it's a

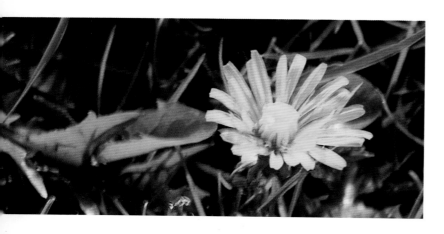

daily herbal formula

Capsules	2 capsules dandelion root 2 capsules burdock root 2 capsules cleavers	◆ Take three times a day with meals
Tincture	1 teaspoon dandelion root 1 teaspoon burdock root 1 teaspoon cleavers	◆ Take in ½ glass of water three times a day with meals
Extract	20 drops dandelion root extract 20 drops burdock root extract 20 drops cleavers extract	◆ Take in a little water three times a day with meals

great cleansing herb. Its name comes from the French *dent-de-lion*, after leaves which look like a lion's teeth. When it comes to healing they carry the strength of a lion's open mouth. Never underestimate the power of the dandelion.

Traditionally, wise women have always used dandelion for cooling fevers and clearing boils. Eye disorders, diarrhoea, fluid retention, liver problems and heartburn can all be treated with dandelion. Knowledge of one of dandelion's strongest effects has been passed on by children from generation to generation. It is disguised in the tale 'if you pick a dandelion you will wet the bed'. This herb is a powerful diuretic. One of the problems associated with many prescribed pharmaceutical diuretics is they can cause important minerals such as potassium to be flushed out of the system. By contrast, however, dandelion is rich in many mineral salts – iron, silicon, magnesium, sodium, potassium, zinc, manganese, copper and phosphorus. They come packaged in a synergistic balance that replaces any minerals lost through increased urination.

tap the root

Dandelion's cleansing effects go even further. The bitter compounds in its root stimulate the flow of bile to aid digestion and boost a sluggish liver. Its content of the vitamin choline gently supports the liver's work – the organ most responsible for clearing wastes, including the elimination of excess hormones such as oestrogens, which can build up to cause reproductive problems in men and women. Dandelion packs a double whammy for PMS: clearing excess hormones and getting rid of water retention at the same time.

All of this makes dandelion an excellent cleansing herb – one which I turn to time and again when my system is feeling overloaded. This is why it plays a starring role in my Herbal Cleanse. But don't miss its cameo roles in the pages on making wonderful salads (see pages 51 and 71) and caffeine (see page 57). Dried dandelion root is easy to come by – loose, in capsules, as a tincture, even in tea bags. Or you can dry your own and grind it in a coffee grinder or with a pestle and mortar.

rich, dark and bitter

I remember children rushing out on to the street when the van from the fizzy drinks factory came visiting, greeting it with far more excitement than the ice-cream seller. They all wanted one thing, rich, dark and bitter – Dandelion & Burdock. Years later I was more than a little surprised to discover that mixing these two herbs makes a wonderful detoxifier. Burdock (*Arctium lappa*) has diuretic and mildly laxative properties which help to remove toxins. Dandelion is rich in potassium, which helps to balance the excretion of fluids. Burdock also contains inulin and the glycoside lappin, which encourage the processing of waste through the kidneys. Together, dandelion and burdock work hard to clear the body through its waste disposal units – the liver, kidneys, skin and colon. Recent research shows that burdock enhances immunity all round. It is one of the safest, most valuable remedies in the world against rheumatic complaints, psoriasis, sciatica and gouty conditions. Burdock's soothing nature can be a real boon to sufferers of eczema, acne and psoriasis too.

burdock bonus for PMS

Burdock can be a blessing for any woman who suffers the sort of PMS that leaves your lower body horrendously heavy as though you have been standing on the same spot for too long. It eases the fluid retention that weighs down legs and its inulin content improves muscle tone in the whole of the lower body. Furthermore, at a time when you are feeling a little frayed anyway, burdock is a gentle and soothing plant friend to use. It takes the rough edges off the natural spring-cleaning process that goes on throughout a menstrual period and 'oils the works' –

stimulating bile secretion and the production of digestive juices to relieve the tummy upsets that come with
PMS and menstruation.

You can take burdock root as a tincture or dried and
powdered. Buy it loose or in capsules. If you are sure you
can identify burdock and don't confuse it with other
similar looking plants, you can also pull it up and dry
your own. Gather the roots of plants at the end of their
first year's growth. Soothing as it may be, burdock packs
a punch. Some herbalists suggest that it is not a good
idea to use it day-in-day-out long-term in tea form as it
is hard to regulate the dose. For the Herbal Cleanse I
find it best to use the tincture, extract, or capsules.

what's grass for the goose

My cats love cleavers (*Galium aparine*). They carry the
tiny round black seeds in through the cat flap hidden
deep in their fur. They then wantonly distribute them
around the carpet so they get stuck to my socks. No
washing machine known to man has ever removed
them. The leaves and stems of cleavers – sometimes
called goose grass – are pale and beautiful, strong and
determined, with little hairs like lush green Velcro, which
grip hard and push the leaves up towards the sky. It is
these parts of the plant that pack the cleansing punch.

Cleavers is a prime mover. It covers the ground with
lightning speed, sweeping away everything in its path.
This is how it works in your body too. Cleavers gets the
lymphatic system moving and strengthens the kidneys,
clearing out wastes, toxicity and infection. With its high
levels of citric acid, rubichloric acid and tannic acid, the
bitter cleavers herb acts as a tonic to the whole system,
stimulating liver function and improving digestion.
Cleavers has a reputation for being cooling to the body.
Traditionally it was used to lower fevers and calm inflammation. Its high mucilage content makes it soothing.
Cleavers could be called a 'man's herb' as it can help urinary tract problems in men and can be useful in the
treatment of an inflamed and enlarged prostate.

Cleavers' soothing quality is one of the major reasons I use it in the Herbal Cleanse. Its gentle cleansing
action can best be described as cool and green, just like
the plant.

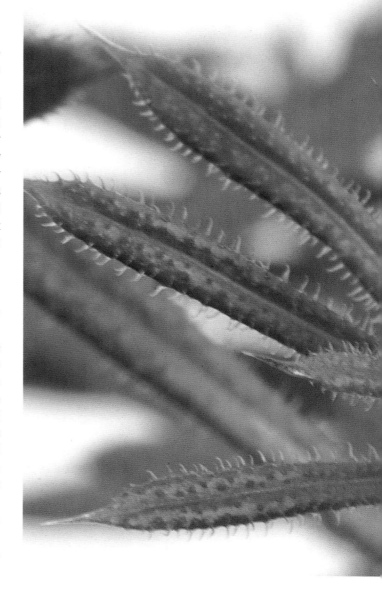

dandelion tea

▶ *2-3 tsp dried dandelion root*
▶ *1 cup water*

Put the dried dandelion root in a pan with the water and
simmer for 15 minutes. Strain, and drink three cups a day.
If you prefer to take a tincture, the dose is 1 teaspoon in
water with meals, or two capsules three times a day.

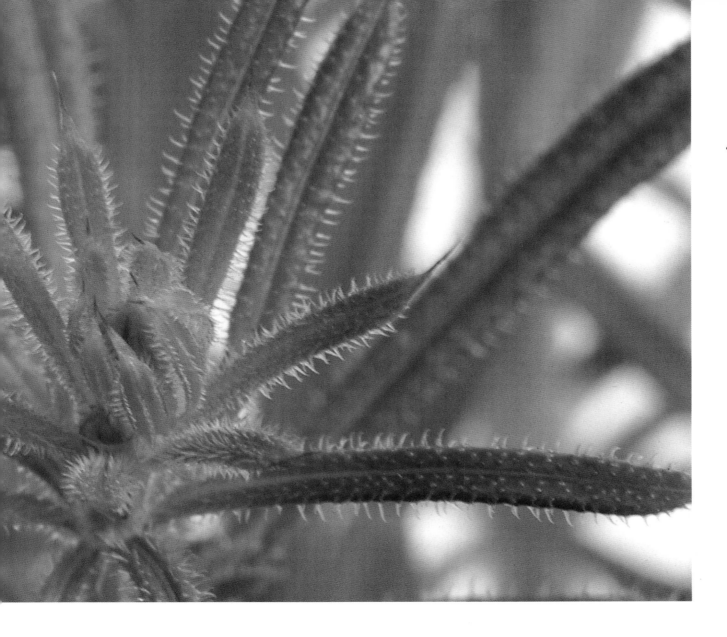

burdock tea

▶ *1 tsp dried burdock root*
▶ *2 cups of water*

Put the dried burdock root into the water in a pan and simmer for 5 minutes. Strain and drink.

cleavers tea

▶ *2-3 tsp dried leaves and stem of cleavers*
▶ *1 cup boiling water*

Pick the cleavers before you see the flowers. Put the dried herb in a tea pot and pour the boiling water over it. Steep for 10-15 minutes. Use three times a day. If you prefer to use a tincture, take ¼-1 teaspoon of tincture in water three times a day with meals.

just do it

I suggest you do this on a Friday so if you need a little extra rest during the first couple of days of the cleanse, you can get it. Now is the time to stop taking in caffeine – tea, coffee, colas, etc – and start drinking more mineral water. Or try out a few herb teas. Make lunch the last 'proper' meal of the day. Eat fresh fruit instead of your evening meal that night. This gives your body an extra 12 hours to get into its elimination. The next seven days of your Herbal Cleanse will follow the plan outlined opposite.

regeneration

During any detox programme it is important to get plenty of rest. Your body's natural elimination processes depend very much on a balance between anabolic and catabolic activities. Anabolic activities are those that build up tissues and repair cells. They won't work properly unless your body's catabolic processes – those involved in breaking down old proteins and eliminating old wastes – are also working well. Taking time out to rest and sleep is really important. Long, gentle walks will help the elimination process. Take a nap in the middle of the day whenever you can and spend more time in bed at night reading, listening to music, or doing anything else that brings you pleasure. It's as simple as that. Take a look at the pages that follow for a few hints and tips on making your detox a fun one. Go for it.

When deciding what to eat during the detox the rule is simple: avoid taking in any foods that might add more toxins – things like coffee and tea, alcohol and convenience foods, like cakes and chocolate. You will also cut out wheat, flour, wheat pasta or anything else made with wheat, as well as all milk products including yoghurt, cheeses, cream, milk or anything made from them. A little butter is OK since it is a fat and it is milk proteins that cause problems.

Include 1-2 tablespoons of pure cold-pressed flax seed oil or better still Udo's Choice – an excellent balance of both Omega 3 and Omega 6 essential fatty acids that must be included in a daily diet – twice a day (see Resources). You can also dress your salads with them or pour them over cooked vegetables (but don't cook with them as heating destroys their goodness). This will ensure that you have adequate essential fatty acids and helps elimination by lubricating the liver and bile ducts. You can use extra virgin olive oil on your salads if you prefer or a mixture of the two.

a note about breakfast

Prunes may not have the sexiest reputation but give prune juice a try, you may be surprised at how useful it is on a detox. Make sure what you buy is not sweetened. Be sure to grind your flax seeds fresh every day to prevent them going rancid, or seal them in an airtight container after grinding and store in the fridge. Keep the packet in the fridge too. Flax seeds are also a gentle laxative as they are high in oil and rich in fibre. They act as a lubricant on the lower intestine.

make a friend of fennel

Fennel has the prettiest leaves of any herb I know. They are as light and fluffy as ostrich feathers yet when you look closely you discover they are a rich dark green. It is the little beige seeds that hold the plant's secrets for healing. Women throughout the ages in Europe hung bouquets of fennel leaves over their door on Midsummer's Eve to protect the home from witchcraft. I have always figured this was because no hideous hag could bear to look upon anything so beautiful.

There are many varieties of fennel and each one is a little different. The most common medicinal variety is

the herbal cleanse

Breakfast	◆ Glass of prune juice and flax seeds (see below)
	◆ Raw fruit
	◆ 100% rye toast if you're still hungry
	◆ Cup of fennel tea (see overleaf)
	◆ Herbal formula (see page 42)
Mid-morning	◆ Cup of fennel tea
Lunch	◆ Fresh fruit or a glass of fruit juice
	◆ An exuberant raw salad (see page 51) made with the freshest organic vegetables you can find, dressed with extra virgin olive oil and lemon or vinegar plus herbs and spices. Eat your salad with home-made soup or a jacket potato or a selection of steamed vegetables
	◆ Herbal formula
Mid-afternoon	◆ Cup of fennel tea
Dinner	◆ Another sensuous salad with a piece of grilled or steamed fish, or perhaps chicken breast roasted or wok fried, an omelette, or some toasted tofu with brown rice or steamed vegetables
	◆ Cup of herb tea or coffee substitute
	◆ Herbal formula
Before bed	◆ Cup of camomile tea (see below) or a good relaxing herbal mixture containing hops, lettuce, passionflower, camomile and other calming herbs

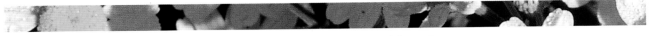

prune juice and flax seeds

▶ *1 tbsp vacuum packed flax seeds or linseeds*
▶ *1 cup prune juice*

Grind the flax seeds or linseeds in a coffee grinder or blender, then blend with the prune juice. Let it stand for 10 minutes to allow the flax seeds to swell. Follow with a glass of water to smooth its journey through your stomach.

camomile tea

▶ *2 tsp dried camomile flowers*
▶ *1 cup hot water*

Put 2 teaspoons of the dried flowers into a tea pot. Pour a cup of hot water over them. (Increase the quantities proportionately to include dinner guests.) Steep for 15 minutes. Strain and drink. Alternatively, you can find camomile in tea bags in health food stores. Because I don't like the taste of it I mix camomile with peppermint or vervain when I make tea.

the perennial herb *Foeniculum vulgare*. It has an enduring reputation as an appetite suppressant. Culpeper wrote that fennel broth made fat people thin, and further back in the Middle Ages parishioners secretively munched fennel seeds at the back of the church during long sermons and on fast days. Throughout history it has been used as a breath freshener, as a gargle for sore throats and coughs, as an eyewash, and as a remedy to expel worms.

Fennel soothes and calms the gut thanks to its volatile oil content, which not only stimulates the production of enzymes but also helps relax spasm in the digestive tract. Culpeper recommended it for hiccoughs and it has a mean reputation for getting rid of indigestion and wind. Fennel seeds are a common ingredient in Indian food and are offered to chew after a meal to soothe digestion and sweeten the breath. Fennel is also a gentle diuretic. Its ability to increase urine flow while soothing digestion makes it the perfect tea to drink throughout the Herbal Cleanse. Three times during the day you will be drinking a cup of fennel tea. Fennel is not only delicious it also soothes the stomach and relieves flatulence – an unfortunate, if occasional, by-product of detoxification. It also suppresses appetite and helps keep you from reaching for the mid-afternoon chocolate bar.

fennel tea

▶ *1 tsp fennel seeds*
▶ *2 cups boiling water*

Use only the seeds. You can buy them loose from health food stores and Indian supermarkets and as fennel tea bags. Steep the seeds in the boiling water for 5 minutes and then strain. Drink this hot immediately. Or make a whole pot, put it in the fridge and have it cold later. If you like a stronger flavour, bruise the seeds first.

Caution:
Fennel stimulates the uterus so avoid drinking fennel tea during pregnancy. Do not give fennel oil to babies or children as it can cause throat spasms.

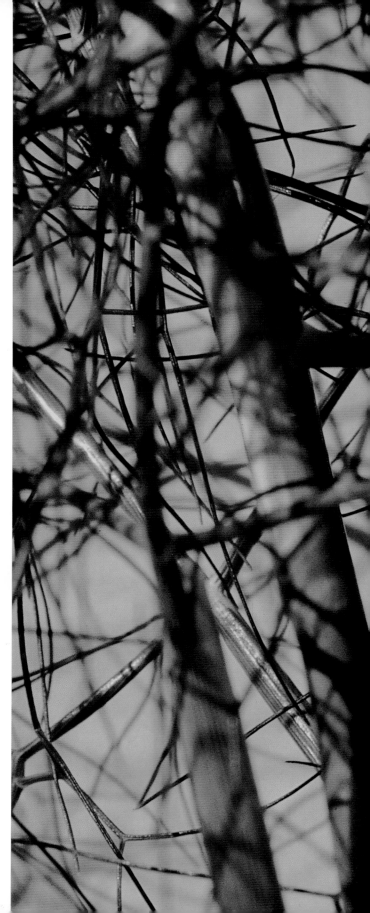

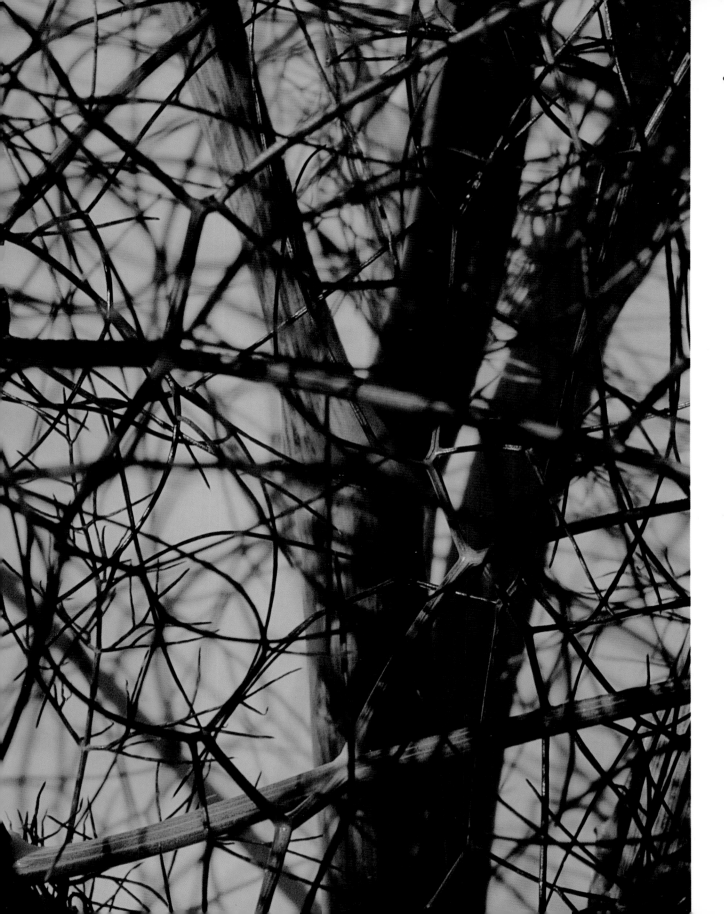

just do it

cleansing foods

foods to choose

- Fresh whole fruits – preferably organic: apples, bananas, cherries, grapefruit, lemons, melons, oranges, etc

- Fresh vegetables both raw and cooked and organically grown if possible – jacket potatoes, artichokes, beetroot, carrots, peas, onions, tomatoes, cabbage, etc

- Fresh, unsweetened fruit and vegetable juices

- Sprouted seeds and grains – mung, lentil, alfalfa, radish, soy, etc

- Small amounts of fresh raw nuts, sunflower, sesame and pumpkin seeds

- Good quality lean meat, poultry (preferably organic) and fresh fish

- Whole grain cereals from oat porridge and brown rice to buckwheat

- 100% wheat-free bread such as rye-bread

- Tofu

- Organic brown rice

- Extra virgin olive oil, Udo's Choice, flax seed oil

- Seasoning: herbs, seaweed, Marigold Swiss Vegetable Bouillon (see Resources), cider vinegar, salt flakes

- Soya milk, rice or almond milk in tea or coffee substitute if you can't face them without milk

- Raw honey, maple syrup, stevia

- Spring water

foods to lose

- Coffee, tea, colas and soft drinks

- Alcohol

- Dairy products – milk, cheese, eggs

- Wheat and wheat products – including cakes and biscuits: read packaging carefully

- Convenience foods of any kind, from breakfast cereals and microwave snacks to TV dinners

- Margarines, cooking oils that are not cold-pressed, hydrogenated oils, and anything containing them

- Processed grain foods

- Processed desserts of any kind, even tinned fruit

- Artificial colourings or flavourings

- Cigarettes and drugs of any kind

- Packaged sauces and dressings

- Sugar

sensuous salads

It is easy to make delicious salads. You will need plenty of the crunchiest, tastiest ingredients, a pretty bowl, some fresh herbs if you can find them and a sunny disposition. I get tired of people telling me that they would eat more salads but they don't have time to go to all that trouble. It takes me all of 10 minutes to make, dress, and serve a salad for four people that looks wonderful, tastes delicious, and makes a whole meal.

The secret of good salad making is this: shop for good fresh ingredients once or twice a week. Wash your salad vegetables as soon as you get them home and put them into storage bins in the fridge. Then whenever you want a salad just take a few bins out of the fridge, pick up a sharp knife and start chopping. I make my salads using a piece of equipment called a mandolin. It is basically a V-shaped blade with plastic attachments that slot on to it for chopping, slicing and grating. You can't beat the speed and perfection with which it slices up vegetables but it's very sharp so take care not to shred your fingers along with the cabbage. Every good salad consists of a base, a body and a wonderful seasoning:

the base
See what is available locally and try sliced, chopped or shredded: Chinese leaves, mustard and cress, rocket (my favourite), tender young spinach, watercress, radiccio, cos lettuce, little gem, red cabbage, endive, lamb's lettuce, young dandelion leaves or fresh pale chicory.

the body
Add to the base whatever else looks good to give your creation body: sliced fennel, chopped or grated carrot, mangetout, grated apple, red onion, chopped spring onions, a small bunch of grapes, sliced button mushrooms, diced tomato, radishes, sweet peppers, diced avocado, grated beetroot, chopped celery.

the finishing touches
◆ Top with a few toasted sunflower seeds, pumpkin seeds, or cashew nuts.
◆ Dress with a drizzle of cold pressed extra virgin olive oil or Udo's Choice (see Resources), lemon or orange juice, or maybe some balsamic vinegar.

◆ A spoonful of clear honey and a dab of wholegrain mustard, or a little grated ginger or crushed garlic can be fun.
◆ Top it off with a flourish of freshly ground black pepper.
◆ I sometimes use the simplest salad dressing imaginable – olive oil or Udo's Choice, lemon juice, a generous dash of Worcestershire sauce and salt flakes – all added direct to the salad itself. Fantastic!

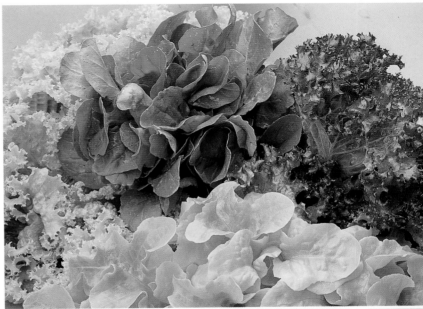

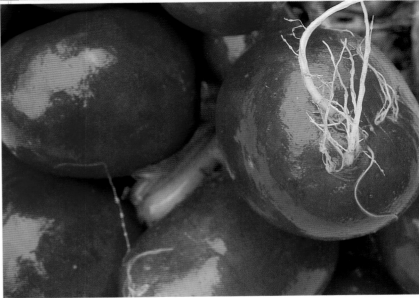

help when you need it

Begin any detoxification programme and your body starts throwing off wastes with great abandon ...

But losing wastes in this way can lead to a few uncomfortable symptoms. You may find your tongue and teeth take on a film that tastes unpleasant for instance. You may have a headache (especially if you are a heavy coffee drinker). You may also feel a little under the weather, even a bit nauseous. A very few people even run a mild fever in the first couple of days. Any of these symptoms – and they by no means occur in every case – are simply a sign that the detox is working. Rejoice. These cleansing reactions quickly pass. Ways to help relieve the most common reactions are given in the table below.

There are lots of things you can do to support elimination and ease symptoms. For a start, drink lots of water during (and after) your detox. When the body's water level gets too low your kidneys don't work efficiently; then the liver has to take on too much of the cleansing work on its own. If you tend to retain water this is often because you don't drink enough so your body tries its best to hold on to the water there is to dilute any toxicity in your tissues. The kidneys and intestines eliminate roughly six glasses of water a day and two are released through the skin.

Here is a simple formula for working out the ideal quantity of water to drink each day for maximum energy. Divide your current weight in kilos by 8 (e.g. 58 kilos divided by 8 = 7.25). Round the figure up (to 8) and that is the number of glasses of water you need a day. This is just a base calculation of course – you will probably need to take in more when exercising or on a hot day.

cleansing reactions

The most common cleansing reactions are headaches, sleeplessness and emotional imbalance. If you have a headache, go and lie down in a quiet, dark room if you can and dab a tiny drop of essential oil of peppermint on your temples and on the back of your neck. Be very careful not to get it into your eyes as it burns. And console yourself with the knowledge that your headache is temporary and wonderful – if uncomfortable – proof that the cleansing process is working.

herbal helpers

To clear a headache	◆ Drink a cup of herb tea such as peppermint, camomile, lemon balm, willow bark. The caffeine in green tea may also help by constricting blood vessels.
For blissful sleep	◆ Drink a cup of camomile or passionflower tea. ◆ Try 10-20 drops of tincture of either valerian or passionflower in water, or take 2 capsules of either valerian or passionflower about 30 minutes before going to bed. (Valerian smells like old socks and isn't a nice tea.)
For emotional comfort	◆ Take 10-20 drops of tincture of motherwort in water three times a day.
For reassurance	◆ Take 10-20 drops of tincture of valerian in water just before bed.

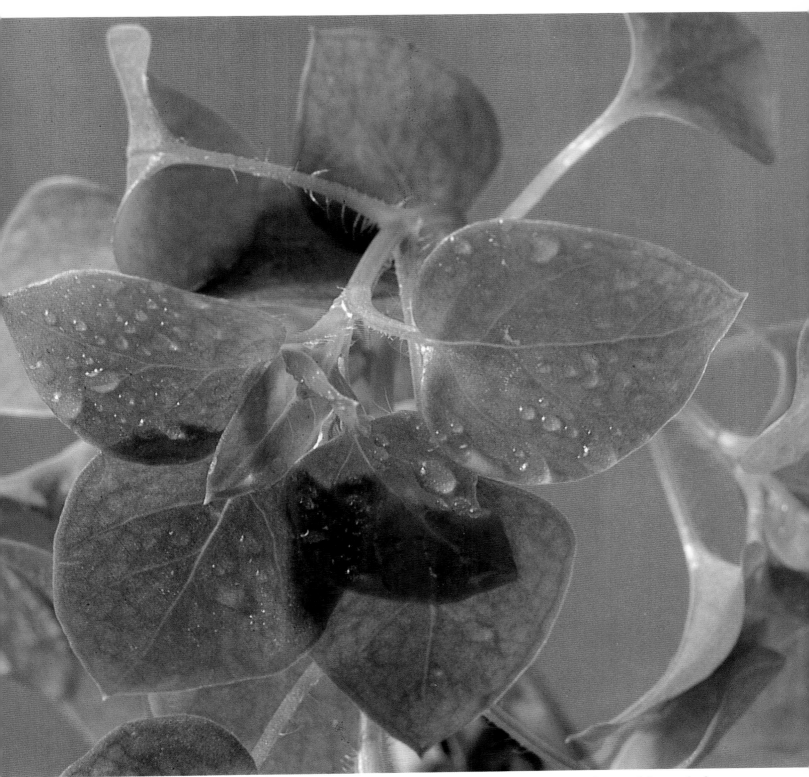
▲ the sight of chickweed raises temperatures in keen gardeners. Yet drink it as a tea and it can banish fever and detox a body.

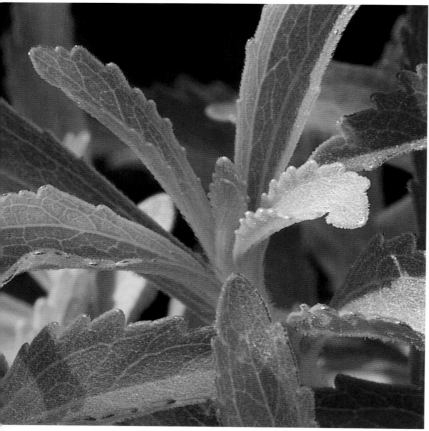

▲ stevia

the brush-off

Almost a third of the body's waste products are eliminated through your skin. Skin brushing is a gentle yet powerful way to stimulate lymphatic drainage and encourage the elimination of wastes. Spend five minutes a day, before your bath, brushing your skin all over with a natural bristle dry brush. Begin at the tips of your shoulders and cover your whole body (except the head) with long smooth strokes over the shoulders, arms and trunk in a downwards motion, then upwards over the feet, legs and hips. You need only go over your skin once for it to work.

The most amazing quantity of rubbish can come out of skin that is brushed regularly. Check for yourself by rubbing a damp flannel over your freshly scrubbed body. Hang the flannel up and use it to repeat the process for a few days. You will find the flannel soon smells of the

waste products that have come directly through the skin's surface. Be grateful they are now outside your body and no longer inside!

the psychic detox

Locked away within all the physical rubbish our bodies have been carrying around is a lot of psychic junk – feelings of anxiety, insecurity and guilt for instance. They can suddenly come to the surface during a detox. They too may be flushed away with the toxins. In the meantime, taking tincture of motherwort or valerian can make you feel better. Repeat the dose three times a day for a few days until you are feeling comfortable again. You can also use soothing essential oils in an oil burner or diffuser to help your mood, or run a bath and put a few drops of essential oil into the running water.

sweeter than sugar

If you have a sweet tooth, you should know about stevia, which you can grow in your garden in summer. It has leaves thirty times sweeter than sugar. Yet it boasts only 1 calorie per ten leaves. It is delicious and easy to use as a sweetener. Stevia is native to South America and is used for diabetics. But you don't have to be diabetic to enjoy its blessings. You can also buy stevia in extract form. Use only a drop or two, however, for this herb is so sweet you will not be able to handle it if you use any more. You can add it to teas, use it in baking, or simply suck on a leaf whenever you feel the need for something sugary.

essential comfort

For feelings of safety	◆ Put a few drops of vanilla essential oil in an essential oil diffuser or 2 drops in the bath
For soothing frayed nerves	◆ Put a few drops of lavender essential oil in an essential oil diffuser or 2 drops in the bath

goldenrod ▶

go for gold

Goldenrod (*Solidago virgaurea*) draws the eye like an actress in a spotlight. It gets all the attention its vivid gold colour demands, and not just because folk tales tell that it points towards hidden gold either. Diuretic, antiseptic and anti-inflammatory, this bold and dazzling plant works with great gentleness to cleanse and clear the urinary system of irritations. It can even soothe mucous membranes ravaged by hayfever. Goldenrod is also my favourite plant for clearing the water logging that comes from fatigue and jet travel. For water logging you can use goldenrod, fresh or dried, and drink it three times a day. Or take ½-1 teaspoon three times a day in water.

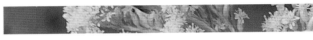

goldenrod tea

▶ *25 g (1oz) fresh flowers of goldenrod or 1 tsp goldenrod leaves*
▶ *600 ml (1 pint) boiling water or 1 cup boiling water*

Steep the fresh flowering tops in boiling water for 10 minutes and strain. Or use the fresh leaves steeped in a cup of hot water for 10 minutes and strain. You can also pour a cup of boiling water over 2-3 teaspoons of the dried herb. Steep for 10-15 minutes and strain.

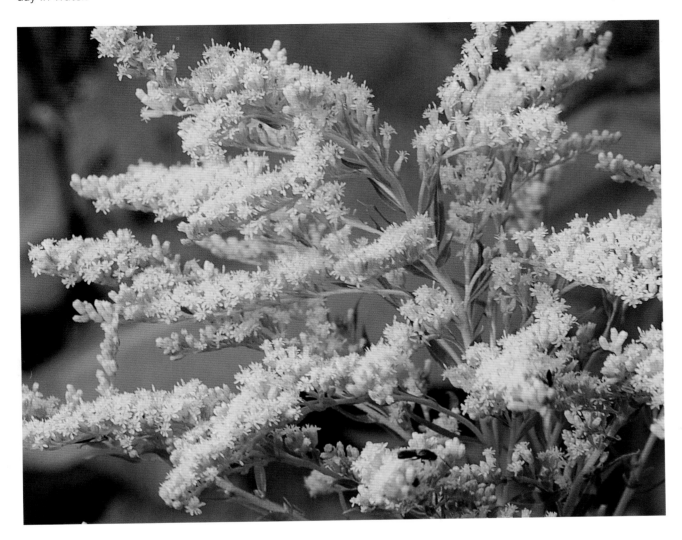

more than a garnish

I've never been quite sure why there is that little pile of parsley sitting atop a restaurant meal but I'm always pleased to see it. Wise women herbalists use parsley (*Petroselinum crispum*) to treat liver and kidney problems, for jaundice and asthma, and to improve digestion. It is an excellent cleanser rich in vitamins A and C, several B vitamins, calcium and iron. In fact, this little green bundle is one of the richest sources of vitamin C we have.

Parsley has diuretic properties as well. It contains two important plant chemicals, myristicin and apiole, believed to increase the flow of blood to the kidneys and therefore to help cleanse the body. Tea made from fresh parsley has a light, wholesome green taste. It seems to make things better from the moment it touches your tongue.

life after caffeine?

'Give up tea and coffee? But that could be the biggest shock to my system since birth!' We start on caffeine in colas and fizzy drinks as children, and take up our parents' tea drinking habits somewhere in our teens. By the time we hit adulthood we end up with a mean coffee habit that began socially and somehow ran away with us. Coffee's the biggest crutch many people have. Don't worry, you need only quit drinking it for a few days. But be aware of how your energy soars four to five days into the Herbal Cleanse. You could well find you prefer a caffeine-free/energy-rich life-style afterwards too.

Too much caffeine has been linked to insomnia, nervousness and anxiety, raised blood pressure, heart palpitations, headaches, irritable bowel syndrome, infertility, fibrocystic breast disease, miscarriage, energy slumps and irritability. More than a small cup or two of coffee a day is likely to give you problems in the long-term.

With the fabulous array of herb teas suitable for all needs and occasions it's a wonder we drink so much tea and coffee at all. Once you make the break away from ordinary tea and coffee you will be amazed at your increased energy and the ease with which you breeze through stressful situations. If drinking herb tea seems like a poor excuse for your beloved cuppa, let me see if I can change your mind. There is one rule to apply to

parsley tea

▶ *2-3 sprigs fresh parsley or 1 tsp dried parsley*
▶ *1 cup boiling water*

Crush the sprigs of fresh parsley or use the dried parsley and pour the boiling water over it. Allow to steep for 5-10 minutes, strain, and drink. You can use parsley tea two or even three times a day.

Caution:
It is OK to eat parsley as a garnish during pregnancy but drinking lots of parsley tea is not a good idea as it may overstimulate the uterus.

green tea

▶ *1-2 tsp dried green tea*
▶ *1 cup boiling water*

Put the dried green tea (you can buy it by the packet in health-food stores) in a tea pot and pour the boiling water over it. Allow it to steep for 5 minutes and drink neat or mixed with peppermint.

Caution:
Green tea contains a high proportion of fluoride. If you are concerned about consuming high quantities of fluoride, drink the antioxidant tea on page 137.

herb teas. Experiment. Mix them together and add some flavourings. Look for boxes of herbal teas in the shops and then make your own using the same mixtures. You will soon wonder what you ever saw in that bland brown stuff you used to drink all day long. For example, try throwing in a couple of cloves, or using a cinnamon stick as a stirrer. Sprinkle with nutmeg, drop in a little honey, or add a drop or two of pure vanilla essence to the final mixture. Delicious!

green is great

If you are a confirmed tea drinker, try green tea. It comes from the same plant as black tea, but rather than allowing the leaf to ferment – which effectively eliminates most of its health benefits – green tea is made by simply lightly steaming the freshly cut leaf. It offers great antioxidant protection against ageing and degeneration, gobbles up free-radicals and boosts your body's own antioxidant defences. Although green tea also contains caffeine, it tends not to stimulate and irritate like a cup of tea or coffee. Best of all, it tastes great. I like it on its own or mixed with peppermint.

send in the chicory

There are several coffee substitutes on the market. Some are even palatable. Those that combine chicory and dandelion are particularly good as they support liver function. Chicory builds energy over time rather than producing the roller coaster energy ups and downs of coffee. Or if you prefer you can make a coffee substitute yourself at home. Try out your own combinations to find the one for you. One of mine is given below to get you going – experiment with your own mixtures.

fresh and minty

Peppermint tea is a wonderful pick-me-up. In the morning it can help you get going. It also stimulates the bowels – something coffee drinkers often use as their excuse for a shot of caffeine first thing. Peppermint's clean taste refreshes the mouth and clears the head, making it a good choice for the mid-afternoon slump which office workers dread. You can buy good quality peppermint tea bags in any supermarket. Keep a packet nearby while you work.

chicory combination

▶ 2 tsp dandelion root
▶ 2 tsp chicory root
▶ 2 tsp burdock root
▶ 2.5 cm (1 in) piece of liquorice
▶ 5 cm (2 in) piece of cinnamon stick
▶ dried orange peel
▶ dried ginger root

Put the whole lot – or half quantities if you like your coffee weak – into a coffee filter machine as if you were making a pot of coffee. Allow it to brew and then drink hot with rice milk or soya milk and a blob of honey if you like. Or combine the ingredients, grind them in a coffee grinder and keep the mix in the fridge. Then simmer 1 teaspoon at a time in a cup of water for 15 minutes, strain and drink hot.

peppermint tea

▶ 3-4 tsp fresh peppermint or 1-2 tsp dried peppermint
▶ 1 cup boiling water

Put the peppermint in a tea pot and pour the boiling water over the top. Allow to steep for 10 minutes, strain and drink. Or dunk a tea bag in a cup of hot water and leave in until it tastes just right.

Caution:
Do not drink too much peppermint tea if breastfeeding as it can reduce the flow of milk.

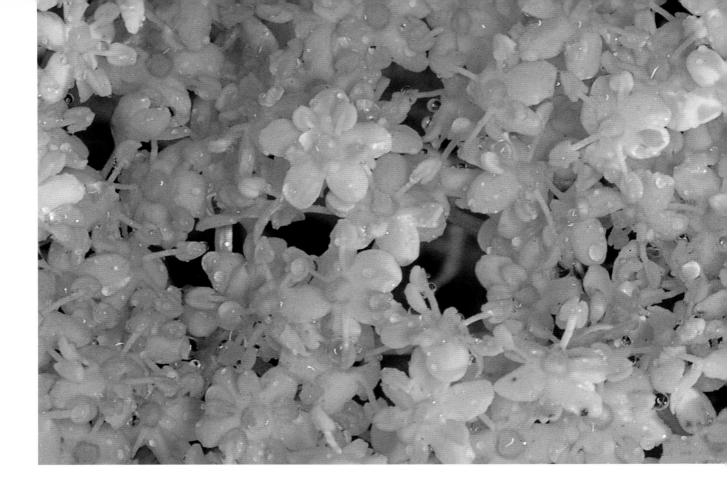

medicine chest tree

Elderflowers are delicate as a bride's veil and they belong to one of the most useful plants I know. Historically, the elder tree (*Sambucus nigra*) was grown outside houses to deter witches, but its uses far exceed banishing the evil eye. In fact, the elder tree has earned itself a reputation as the 'one plant medicine chest'. Elderflowers boast valuable compounds like flavonoids, mucilages and tannins. They are useful in combating the fever and mucus brought by a cold. They are also great just after a cold or flu to help get rid of lingering symptoms for they can help break up mucus stored in the body, allowing it to be more easily eliminated.

People from Denmark believe that the elder holds a spirit called the elder-tree mother, who will forever haunt whomever cuts the tree down. In Britain, cutting any part of an elder traditionally required that you wear a hat and kneel before the plant to ask its permission before doing so.

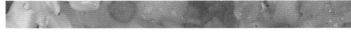

queen of the bubbles

▶ *Boil 4½ litres (8 pints) water*
▶ *Dissolve 450 g (1 lb) golden granulated sugar in the hot water. Let it cool, and add:*
▶ *2 large sliced lemons*
▶ *2 tablespoons of white wine or cider vinegar*
▶ *7 heads of elderflowers, heads down.*

Leave your champagne covered in a stainless steel, crockery, or plastic container for 24 hours. Strain through cheese-cloth or muslin and pour into a clean – preferably sterilized – bottle with a cork (don't use bottles with sealed lids as this champagne is so exuberant it has been known to explode). Store in a cool place and it will be ready to drink when fizzy – in about 2 weeks.

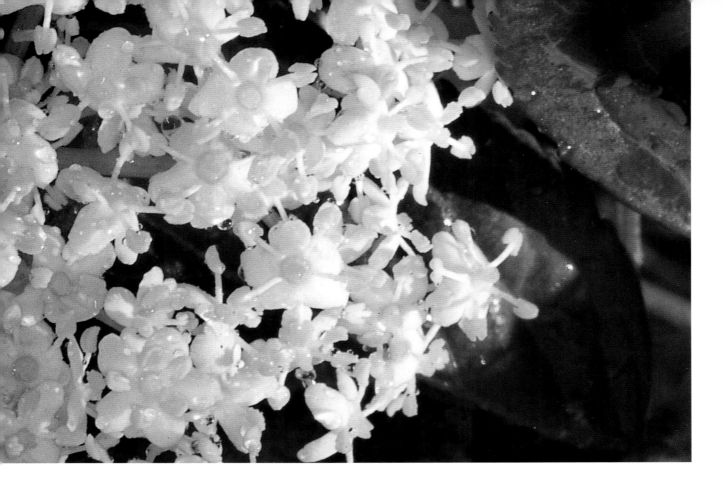

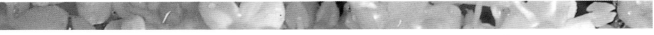

elderflower tea

▶ *2 tsp dried elderflowers*
▶ *1 cup boiling water*

Put the dried elderflowers in a tea pot and pour the boiling water over them. Cover and allow to steep for 15-20 minutes. Strain and drink three times a day. Always pick the flowers when the sun has dried the dew from them.

elderflower punch

▶ *3-4 handfuls fresh elderflowers, removed from branch*
▶ *1 litre (2½ pints) fruit juice*
▶ *1 handful fresh mint leaves*

This is one of my favourite recipes for summer given to me by a very dear friend, Dr Barbara Latto. Put the fresh elderflowers into the fruit juice. Then add the mint leaves – I use pineapple mint, apple mint, spearmint or whatever is growing in abundance – and let the mixture steep cold in the fridge over night. Strain, add carbonated water to taste and serve with a sprig of fresh mint.

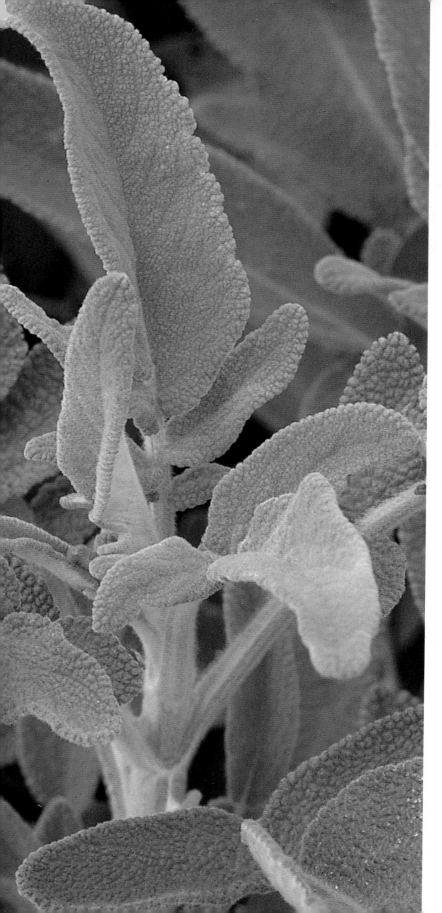

stress buster

Nettle tea is for those moments when you think your head is going to burst. Cool and green it boosts your energy yet calms you at the same time. Such is the synergy our plant friends convey.

the sage wind-down

Sage is one of my favourite herbs. I grow it in the garden and hang bunches tied with ribbon to dry from my kitchen ceiling. Then I reach up and grab a bundle whenever I want tea. Put your feet up and sip sage tea at the end of a long day's work or a trip around the shops. Rich in the calming minerals magnesium, calcium and zinc, sage soothes frayed nerves and levels out emotional mood swings. Sage is also a good tea to reach for if you have a tension headache accompanied by a 'knot' in the stomach. It calms a disturbed stomach and contains saponins that ease pain in the head.

nettle tea

▶ *1-3 tsp dried nettle leaves*
▶ *1 cup boiling water*

Put the dried nettle leaves in a tea pot and pour the boiling water over them. Allow to steep for 10 minutes, strain and drink. If you are going to pick and dry your own nettle leaves, pick them when young and tender and their stinging hairs are not yet fully formed.

sage tea

▶ *1 tsp dried sage*
▶ *1 cup boiling water*

Put the sage in a tea pot and pour the boiling water over the top. Allow to steep for 10 minutes, strain and drink.

Caution:
Do not drink sage tea if you are pregnant as it may cause contractions of the uterus.

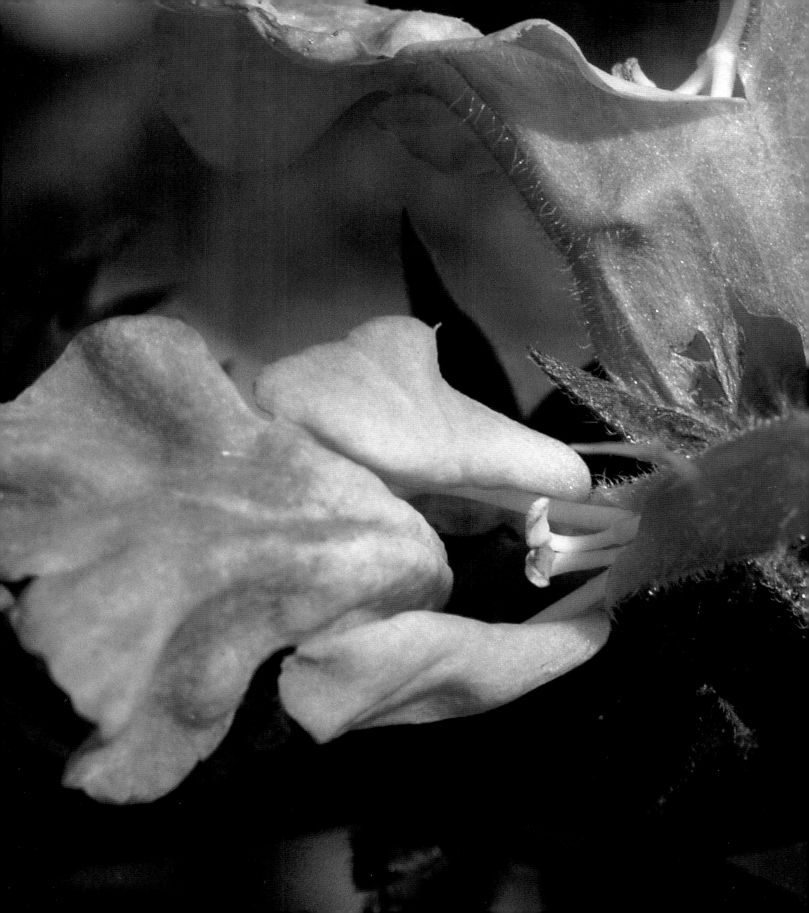

freedom from cigarettes

If you want to give up smoking but don't know where to turn, there's help at hand. Start with the Herbal Cleanse. It will help eliminate a lot of nicotine and other rubbish from your system. The Herbal Cleanse will also give you a psychological boost. Once you have cleaned out your body, even if you smoke during the cleanse, you are likely to feel less like lighting up. There are also lots of specific herbs that can help any smoker to become an ex-smoker.

But before you give up nicotine be familiar with all the things you can do to ease cleansing reactions. Make sure you have everything you might need to hand. Put time aside for yourself to have rests, baths, long walks – whatever you need. And congratulate yourself on deciding to do something positive about your addiction now instead of putting it off again.

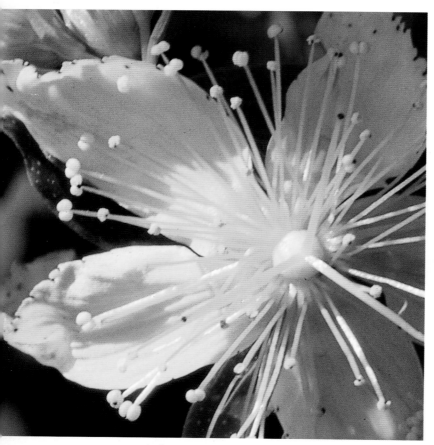

▲ st john's wort

ease your mind

Nicotine has a way of suppressing difficult emotions. When you stop smoking they tend to rush back to the surface almost the way physical symptoms appear when you do a detox. They are trying to clear themselves from your system. Herbs can help make the process more graceful – especially St John's wort. Often called 'nature's Prozac' this plant can take the raw edges off your emotions so you can deal with them more easily as they surface. Take ½-1 teaspoon of St John's wort tincture in water three times a day (see also pages 117-18).

chew away your cravings

Many smokers long for the taste of tobacco. Try chewing on a small piece of dried ginseng root, about the size of your little finger nail. It has a taste quite unlike anything else yet satisfies the mouth in the same way that tobacco does. Ginseng is also famed for strengthening your ability to deal with stress. Buy the best quality you can find (see Resources).

knock nicotine on the head

Skullcap is used to treat drug and alcohol addiction. It can help with all sorts of cravings. Its calming effect is a real blessing to smokers who fear they will no longer be able to deal with stress. Simply taking time out to make a herbal tea instead of fretting over what you continually worry about can help break the habit.

skullcap tea
▶ *2 tsp dried skullcap*
▶ *1 cup boiling water*

Put the dried herb into a tea pot and pour the water over it. Allow to steep for 5 minutes. Strain and drink. Alternatively, whenever you feel that you can't wind down at the end of the day, add 2 teaspoons of dried camomile to your skullcap tea and sip it slowly. This little gem can also help you to sleep.

some like it hot

Submerging your body in warm water is not only relaxing, it also helps ease any niggling cleansing reactions such as headaches or irritability. Here are three methods I particularly like. If any of the baths feel uncomfortable, don't do them, instead get out and perhaps try again in a few days. Never force yourself to endure anything you think is good for you if your instinct says no.

Heat can do a lot to improve your circulation, elimination and mood. According to European experts in hydrotherapy, controlled overheating of the body increases the rate of metabolic processes and acts as a stimulus to the nervous system and the glands. This creates a feeling of mental calm and physical vitality. Artificially induced perspiration is one of the best ways to deep cleanse the body. But never take a heat treatment if you are unwell, suffer from a respiratory ailment or heart disease, or already have a fever.

heat bath treats

To soothe irritability	◆ Add 2 drops of camomile or lavender essential oil as the bath is running
To calm nervous anxiety	◆ Make a bath bag (see page 128) containing ½ cup each of dried camomile flowers and lavender
To ease a tension headache	◆ Make a bath bag containing ½ cup each of dried valerian and peppermint

chill-out baths

Gentle cleanse	◆ 2 cups strong fennel tea (see page 45)
Medium cleanse	◆ 2 cups cider vinegar poured under running water
Strong cleanse	◆ 2 cups each of sea salt and baking soda

Heat baths are simple. Keep the water temperature at about 40-43°C (104-110°F), just a few degrees above normal body temperature. Take a water thermometer (the kind mothers use for baby baths) into the bath with you. Check the temperature every few minutes, topping up with more hot water when necessary. Lie in the bath for 15-20 minutes with all but your head immersed. Get out quickly, wrap yourself in a big towel and lie down in a warm room for 20 minutes.

chill out

Alternatively, get into hot water to draw toxins to the surface of the skin. Then allow the bath to cool (but not uncomfortably so) and the toxins are pulled into the water. A chill-out bath is great just before going to bed.

epsom salts baths

Epsom salts are magnesium sulphate. Both magnesium and sulphate molecules have an ability to leech excess sodium, phosphorus and nitrogenous wastes from the body through the surface of your skin. They also balance the subtle electrical energies in the body to restore emotional equilibrium. This is why athletes use them to relieve muscular pain and why they are wonderful as a way of unwinding during periods of prolonged stress. Epsom salts baths during a detox are great for easing the aches and pains, fatigue or nervousness which sometimes accompany the body's rapid throwing off of waste. When you get out wrap yourself in a towel and lie down for 15 minutes – or better still go to bed.

the balancing bath

▶ *2 cups household grade Epsom salts*
▶ *(available from your local chemist)*

To banish aches and pains, pour the Epsom salts into a blood-heat bath. Immerse yourself for 20-30 minutes, topping up with warm water to maintain a comfortable temperature.

Caution:
You should only take one detox bath a day, and stop taking them if ever you feel they are too much for you.

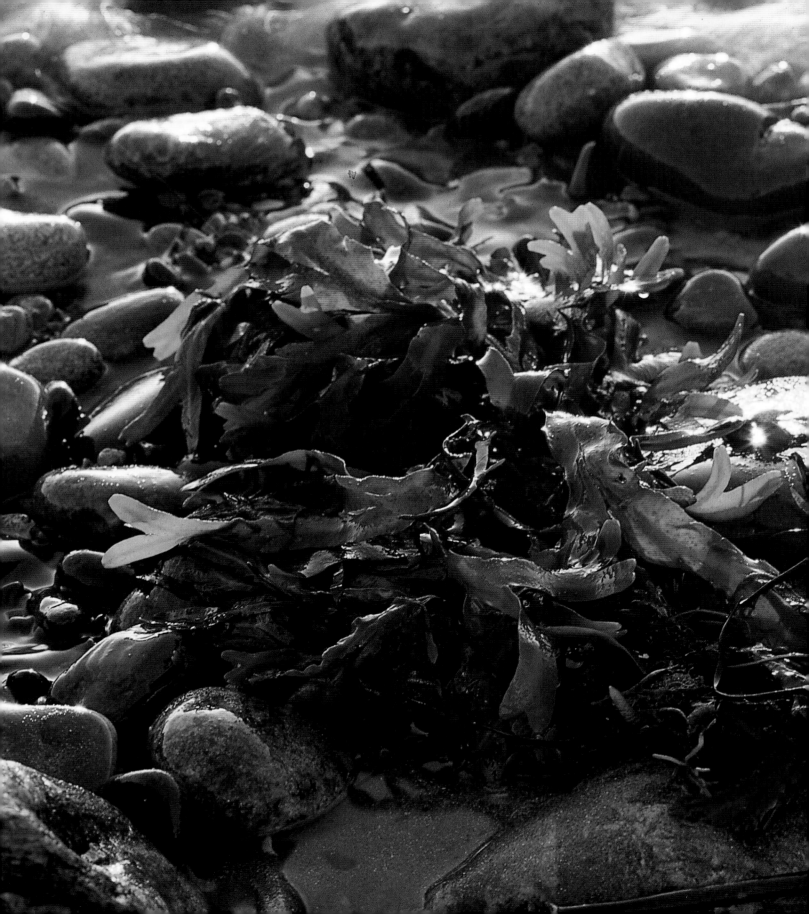

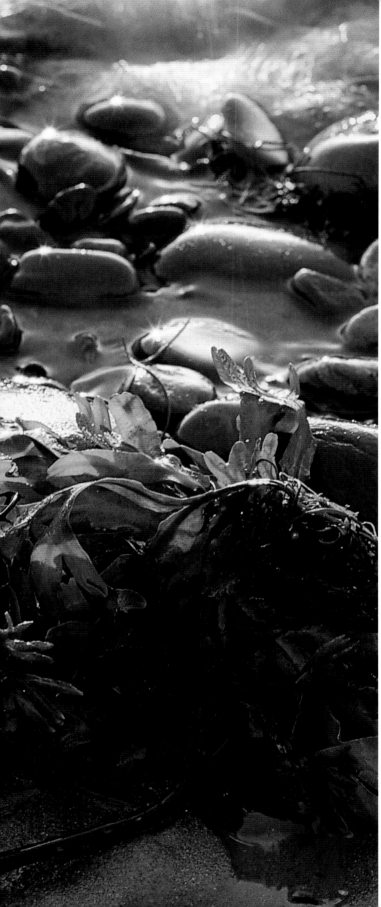

strengthening 3

Detoxification is the first step in renewing your life with herbs. But it is not enough on its own. The modern diet of denatured foods - foods which have been highly processed to turn them into so-called convenience foods - robs the body of many nutrients needed to keep the metabolic processes working properly. You must have specific nutrients - vitamins such as vitamins C and B6 as well as trace elements and minerals like zinc and chromium - to act as co-factors to the enzymes that fuel these metabolic processes.

◄ kelp

natural affinities

The body has a remarkable ability to compensate for what it doesn't have ...

But living on a diet of convenience foods over a period of many years gradually depletes it of vital co-factors and leads to a breakdown in functioning. You will see this occur first in whatever system or organ happens to be your weakest. This, in turn, depends on what you have inherited from your ancestors. One of the best things you can do to strengthen yourself is to call on plants to help restore the levels of minerals and vitamins you may have lost over the years.

Certain herbs directly impact specific organs, systems and metabolic functions: for instance, milk thistle is a powerful strengthener for the liver, shiitake mushrooms for the immune system, hawthorn and olive for the heart, bearberry for the kidneys, marshmallow for the lungs and calendula for the skin. In addition, each plant has a specific spirit or character and it is for this reason that learning to use herbs demands a lot of hands-on experience at deeper levels. In that way you come to know plants in a truly sacred way – not only in your mind but instinctively.

Some herbs act as a tonic on the body. Others disperse stagnant energy or encourage the repair of damage and enhance specific functions. You come to experience this by relating to herbs over a period of time. Before long they become old friends. So touch and smell the plants that attract you. Watch them, listen to them and taste them. They will reveal to you their secrets in a highly personal way – secrets that you can later check against the wise woman traditions and the latest findings in plant research.

Even the flavours of plants can tell you about their use. Sour-tasting plants tend to strengthen the lungs and disperse stagnation in the liver, while bitter-tasting plants like dandelion act as a tonic on the kidneys. Sweet plants, rich in saponins, like liquorice, strengthen soft tissues and balance digestion. Many plants, like garlic, echinacea, dandelion, nettle and olive leaf extract, act as a tonic. They bring strength to the whole organism. Use them when you are well and they can help protect you from illness. If you get sick, getting to know the strengthening herbs can empower your body's natural ability to heal.

power to the liver

When your liver works well so does the rest of your body, for the liver is your body's chemical centre. It is responsible for clearing excess hormones, getting rid of chemicals that could undermine the immune system, and cleansing the toxicity that builds up from too much alcohol, poor food and taking drugs of all kinds. The liver's ability to deep-clean the system helps protect your whole body from premature ageing and degeneration.

The trouble is that the modern world is literally full of potentially dangerous chemicals. We take them in through the chemically fertilized and highly processed foods we eat, through the air we breathe and the water we drink. As a result many livers are overloaded with toxicity and burdened with a volume of work they were never designed to deal with. When your liver becomes toxic you can experience many different symptoms from headaches and itchy eyes to pain in the right side, confusion and depression. Strengthen your liver and you immediately raise your vitality not to mention lifting depressed spirits, even if you have been plagued with them for years. There are all sorts of plants that can help you do this from carrot (yes truly, ordinary carrots) to dandelion, chicory, dang quai or Chinese angelica, liquorice and ginger. Make them a part of your life. The most important liver strengthener of them all is the magnificent milk thistle plant.

▶ echinacea

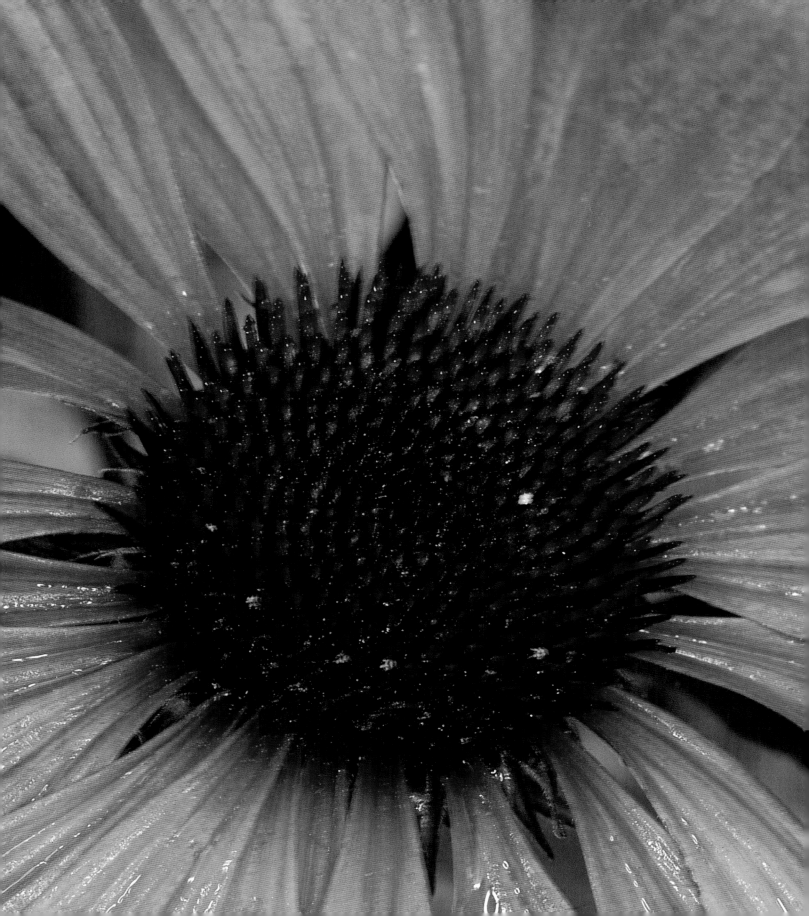

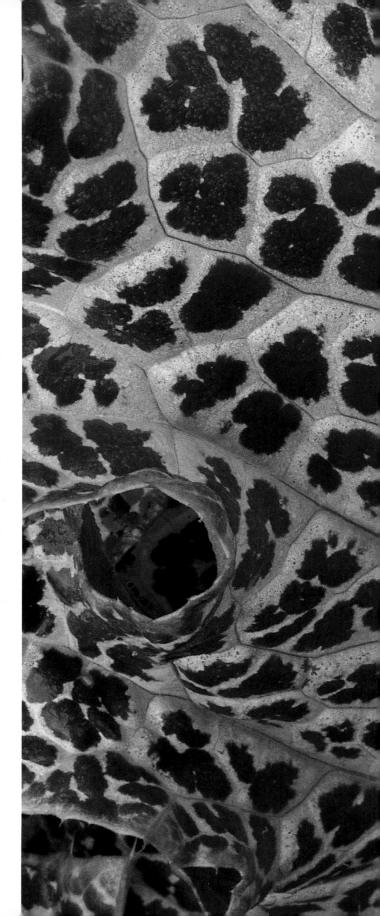

seeds of healing

For more than two millennia, milk thistle (*Silybum marianum*) has been used to strengthen the liver. In large part it is the phytochemical silymarin that appears to be what makes milk thistle so potent a liver protector. Recent studies show that, taken as a preventative herb, it can even help protect the body from damage caused by exposure to highly dangerous – often cancer-causing – industrial toxins in our environment, including carbon tetrachloride.

The lovely dark green milk thistle plant, whose leaves are shot through with milky markings, flowers in early summer and grows to a glorious 180 cm (6 ft) high. The Romans knew about it and used it regularly to counter the effects of their Bacchanal rites. In the nineteenth century, a famous German doctor called Rademacher created a tincture based on milk thistle, which is still used in Europe and bears his name.

The compounds in milk thistle seeds – the most well researched of which is silymarin – not only protect the liver from the damage that alcohol and hepatitis can do, but also actually help regenerate a liver that is already damaged. German doctors, following the protocol set by the prestigious Commission E, use extract of milk thistle as the treatment of choice when dealing with all sorts of chronic liver conditions including hepatitis and cirrhosis – a hardening of the liver tissue often caused by alcoholism which is virtually impossible to treat through conventional medicine.

I love using milk thistle as a prophylactic – that is before I have liver troubles. I use it when I am travelling, for instance, or during periods of prolonged stress since both can put heavy-duty pressure on the liver. You can grow milk thistle (a close relative of the chicory plant) in your garden and harvest it yourself if you like. You can roast and grind the seeds and use them as a coffee substitute. Pick the leaves very young and you can even put them in your salads, but they get unbelievably spiky as they grow and soon become totally inedible. However, when I am using it for healing, milk thistle is one of the herbs I prefer to buy either as a tincture or powdered herb in capsules from a reliable supplier. I also often buy it as a standardized herb so I can be sure of the content of silymarin I am getting. I take milk thistle when I have

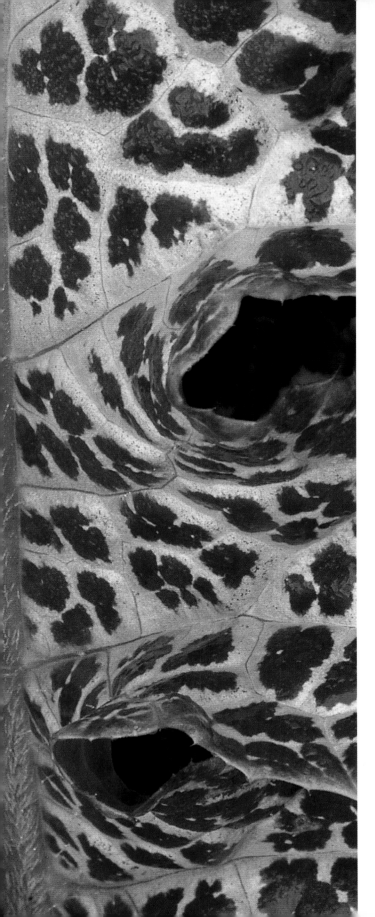

been poisoned by food (or by anything else). You can easily make milk thistle tea, which is great for general protection and to drink every couple of hours when you have a hangover or have been poisoned by something.

the herbalist's prescription for milk thistle

◆ Chronic liver problems: take 2 capsules of the standardized whole herb containing 20-35mg of silymarin or 1 teaspoon of tincture three times a day for six weeks or more.
◆ General protection: from environmental poisoning, as an anti-ageing herb, if you smoke or take alcohol or any kind of drugs (legal prescriptions or illegal): 1 capsule or ½ teaspoon of tincture three times a day.
◆ After exposure to poison: such as carbon tetrachloride or excess alcohol or food poisoning: take 2 capsules or 1 teaspoon of tincture every 3 to 4 hours until the symptoms have subsided.

milk thistle tea

▶ *2 tbsp milk thistle seeds*
▶ *6 cups water*

Bring the water to the boil in a saucepan and then put the seeds in the boiling water. Remove the pan from the stove, cover it and let it sit in a warm place for 30 minutes. Then you can drink the liquid hot or cold. This makes enough for six cups of tea – a whole day's supply if you drink it every 3 to 4 hours. I like to add a bag or two of peppermint tea to the water along with the seed. It improves the flavour and the peppermint itself helps relieve headaches, calms digestion and clears your head.

◀ milk thistle

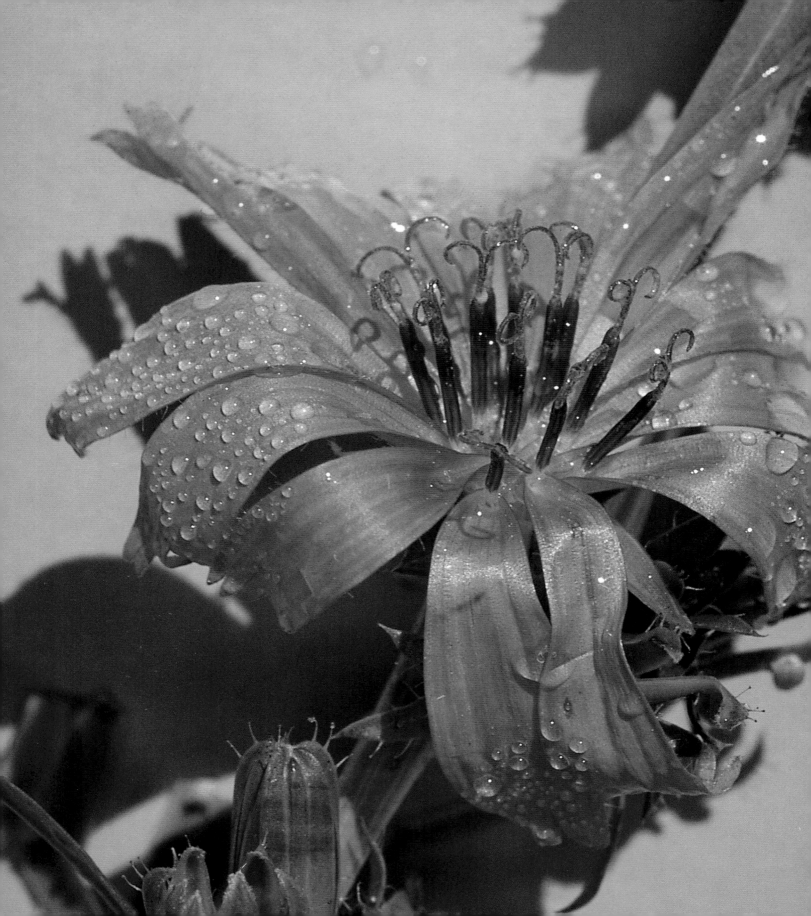

wonder weed

Cultivated in Egypt 5,000 years ago, chicory (*Chichorium intybus*) is a beautiful, gentle plant which pulls a lot of power for healing. It was one of the 75 plants Charlemagne demanded be grown in his own garden because of its beauty and its might. It is now much undervalued. Chicory root is a mild tonic, and has diuretic and laxative properties, which helps strengthen the liver. Just as useful are its leaves. They add buzz to any salad as they are slightly bitter. You can lightly steam them and eat them as a green vegetable too. Chicory is easy to grow. But pick the leaves before the plant flowers as afterwards they become too bitter for most palates.

dandelion

Dandelion is at the top of my list of healthy plants for the liver and digestive system. It is a wonderful overall tonic to strengthen your whole body (see pages 42-3 and 57). Add a few dandelion leaves to fresh vegetable juices in a blender and drink a glass every morning. It is a great way to start the day and, like sea plants, dandelion is rich in vitamins and minerals including iron and potassium. Drink dandelion-root coffee. Toss dandelion leaves in your salads whenever you can – they are free,

abundant and, provided you pick them when they are young, deliciously bitter. The leaves are a natural diuretic. The roots have anti-rheumatic properties and the flowers are rich in lecithin, a nutrient that is useful in protecting the liver. You can even use the white sap from the fresh stem and root as a topical remedy for warts. Make dandelion a part of your day-to-day life and you can grow strong as a lion.

liver strength salad

Just about everything in the salad below not only acts as a tonic for the liver but also strengthens the whole body. In lab experiments, carrots have been shown to protect against liver damage and chemical pollutants. They contain phytochemicals that increase the activity of enzymes involved in the liver's detoxification processes. Turmeric is another great liver protector. Young dandelion leaves and flowers are not only delicious, they strengthen the entire organism.

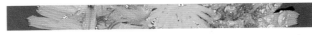

dandelion petal salad

- ▶ *dark green salad leaves, eg rocket, lamb's lettuce*
- ▶ *2.5 cm (1 in) piece ginger, grated*
- ▶ *2 cloves garlic, crushed*
- ▶ *3 carrots, grated*
- ▶ *12 dandelion flowers*
- ▶ *2 tbsp extra virgin olive oil*
- ▶ *juice of 1 lemon*
- ▶ *Worcestershire sauce*
- ▶ *turmeric*
- ▶ *sea salt*
- ▶ *Cajun seasoning*

It is easy to make a great salad that not only tastes delicious but also acts as a tonic for the liver. Fill a bowl with the dark green vegetables and add the ginger, garlic and carrots. Sprinkle with the petals from the dandelion flowers and then add the extra virgin olive oil, lemon juice, a dash of Worcestershire sauce, a pinch of turmeric, some sea salt, a dash of Cajun seasoning and toss. This salad serves 2 to 4.

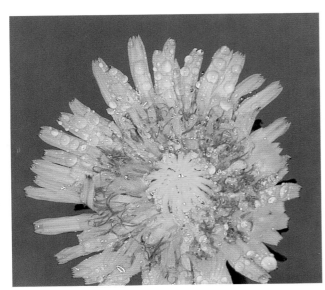

◀ chicory ▲ dandelion

look to the lungs

Strengthen your lungs and you strengthen
your sense of ease in the world ...

In Chinese medicine, lung problems are most often associated with grief. I saw an example of this in my youngest son. He had a wonderful relationship with his nanny, who had been with us until he was eight years old. She felt then that he was too old for her to be useful to him any more and decided to leave. She found separating from this child, whom she so loved, very hard and when he expressed sadness about her going she urged him not to cry. So he swallowed his grief. It soon erupted in asthma attacks. It was not until he felt able to express the grief and let it go that they cleared completely. There are a number of herbs that I use to strengthen the lungs, helping to protect against asthma and bronchitis, sinusitis, coughs and catarrh.

marshmallow means to heal

Its botanical name is *Althaea officinalis* from the Greek *altho* which means 'to heal'. Not only is marshmallow, right, ideal used as an ointment to heal sores and speed wound healing, this lovely plant with flowers rich in flavonoids and mucilage also soothes mucous membrane and strengthens the lungs against attack from exposure to passive smoking and pollution. It also soothes, strengthens and tones the bladder, helping to protect the urinary system from infection. You can make an infusion of marshmallow and drink it three times a day.

elderberry protectors

Long before the coming of vitamin C syrups, wise women used elderberries (*Sambucus nigra*) to strengthen the lungs and protect from winter colds and flu. Elderberry supports the immune system too and is a natural laxative, which is why elderberry tinctures are so useful in detoxifying the body. I recommend taking 1 teaspoon of tincture in a little water three times a day.

roman secrets

In practice Roman camomile (*Anthemis nobilis*), left and its near cousin German camomile (*Matricaria chamomilla*) are practically identical in properties. It is the flowers from these plants that you use either in tea form – drunk a couple of times a day – or as a tincture: 1 teaspoon in half a glass of water before bed each night. They are a gentle but effective way to strengthen both lungs and nervous system against asthmatic attacks in those prone to them. For recipe for camomile tea see page 47.

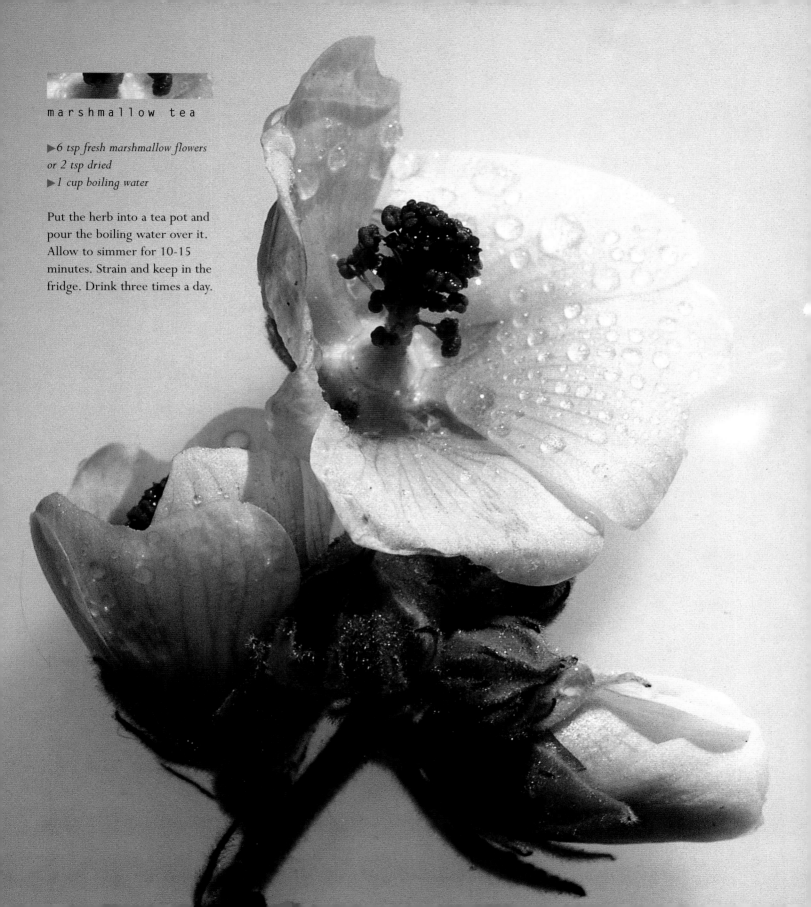

marshmallow tea

▶ *6 tsp fresh marshmallow flowers*
or 2 tsp dried
▶ *1 cup boiling water*

Put the herb into a tea pot and
pour the boiling water over it.
Allow to simmer for 10-15
minutes. Strain and keep in the
fridge. Drink three times a day.

antiviral power

Use plants to strengthen yourself against viral infections and you will end up very strong indeed ...

Viruses are weird things – so small you cannot even see them under a normal microscope. Scientists cannot decide if they are living things or not since they don't eat, use oxygen or eliminate wastes. What they do – in no uncertain terms – is to reproduce once they have infected a susceptible body. Antibiotics are virtually useless against viruses even though some doctors continue to prescribe them.

When it comes to antiviral drugs, these are as scarce as hens' teeth. I can think of only two: acyclovir used against herpes and AZT against AIDS. Yet there are many potent antiviral herbal remedies. Bring them into your life. Many act as a tonic to the whole system. Furthermore, they are useful both for protection and as a means of helping your body clear viral infections when they occur.

garlic earns a medal

When it comes to antiviral and antibacterial power, there is no plant in the world like garlic. Everything that antibiotic drugs can do, garlic does better, safer and cheaper. It may take a little longer but, in the process, using garlic regularly will build your strength and balance your body instead of leaving you exhausted and in a mess as many drugs do after treatment. So make garlic a day-to-day part of your life. Cook with it, prepare garlic vinegars and garlic oils for your salads. Eat chopped garlic on your baked potatoes. Use it any way you can think of. It helps safeguard health and youth.

Garlic is most effective eaten raw and is really enjoyable crushed or minced in salads or pasta. If you worry about the smell, chew a sprig of parsley after your meal

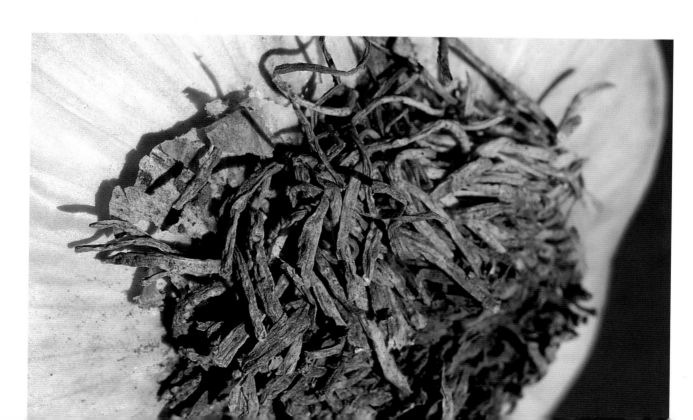

and never drink cheap red wine with garlic. It sours the breath badly. Come to think of it, never drink cheap red wine at all. Take one or two cloves (not bulbs!) of garlic every day in your foods. If you really don't think you can manage two cloves of fresh garlic, make pickled garlic and use it as a condiment.

Hundreds of studies have demonstrated garlic's antimicrobial power. It kills bacteria, viruses, fungi and protozoa. It also has 5,000 years of recorded history of use against illness. Hippocrates recommended garlic for infections. Its folk use is ubiquitous. So powerful is this wonder plant that when penicillin supplies ran out in the Second World War, Russian medics used garlic instead. Famous for its heart benefits, garlic has an ability to reduce high blood pressure.

Recent popular interest in garlic has been increased by the bad publicity given to cholesterol. Garlic decreases levels of the harmful type of cholesterol and can even help prevent blood clots responsible for heart attacks and strokes. A recent Russian study has shown that garlic has a twofold effect on heart disease, having a direct action on the walls of the heart's arteries, and also having a preventative effect at a cellular level. Garlic also boosts immunity, balances blood sugar, helps the liver to deal with toxins and relieves digestive problems. Garlic contains amino acids, vitamins and trace elements, flavonoids, enzymes and dozens of unusual sulphur compounds rarely found in other plants. It is these sulphur compounds that some scientists believe are responsible for garlic's antibacterial, antiviral and antioxidant qualities. Garlic is also one of the greatest natural sources of selenium.

There is no consensus of opinion on what makes garlic so beneficial. According to some studies it is the alliin which is transformed into allicin – a potent antibacterial agent – when garlic is crushed. Manufacturers of garlic supplements are increasingly standardizing their products for alliin and allicin, as well as for total sulphur content and S-allyl cysteine. But arguments still rage as to which of these is the 'active ingredient'. This has made many herbal doctors reject capsules and tablets in favour of raw garlic. Some herbalists believe that garlic's antimicrobial properties are lost through processing.

The debate goes on. I prefer to use whole garlic – and lots of it, too. Buy it fresh, juiced, in tablets, capsules and tinctures. There are plenty of garlic products that don't give off the characteristic odour if you can't handle its smell.

garlic oil

▶ *1 large bulb fresh garlic*
▶ *olive oil*

Mince the garlic and put in the top of a double boiler. Pour in enough olive oil to cover the garlic by an 2.5 cm (1 in) and warm gently for an hour. Cool, strain through muslin or cheesecloth, and keep in a sealed bottle or jar in the fridge. Use it on your salads; it's delicious.

Caution:
Garlic acts as a blood thinner so it is wise not to take with anticoagulant drugs. Taking large daily doses - more than 10 g - can cause stomach irritation or indigestion

pickled garlic

▶ *1 cup water*
▶ *1 cup cider vinegar*
▶ *1 cup soy or Worcestershire sauce*
▶ *1 cup honey*
▶ *lots of garlic*

Combine the water, cider vinegar, soy or Worcestershire sauce and honey in a saucepan and warm to dissolve the honey. Half fill a jar (with a tight-fitting lid) with the mixture and drop in as many peeled cloves of garlic as you have. You need to make sure that the pickling mix covers the garlic so add more of it if needed. Tightly close the lid and keep in the fridge for two weeks before eating. Your pickled garlic will keep for about two months.

chinese wonder plant

Another great immune protector is what the Chinese call huang qi – astragalus. Astragalus is the root of the yellow vetch plant. Unlike many herbs, it actually tastes good. Creamy yellow, it is a favourite among the Chinese for strengthening digestion, overcoming chronic weakness and enhancing wound-healing. Whenever there is a deficiency of life energy, reach for this tonic herb. Astragalus brings deep strength to the immune system. It increases the number and quality of white blood cells used to fight infection. This is why it is often used with HIV and cancer patients whose immune systems have been undermined by chemotherapy or radiation. Research shows it is even effective against the nasty Coxsackie B virus, which is responsible for inflammation of the heart.

On a day-to-day basis, astragalus is especially useful as winter approaches since it can help you ward off flu and colds. Three cups of astragalus tea a day should do the trick (one cup a day for children) so long as you take it consistently every day. Chinese medicine defines ailments as being either 'hot' or 'cold' and herbs as being 'warming' or 'cooling'. Astragalus is a warming herb to be used with 'cold' illnesses, and unless you know what kind of cold or flu you have don't take it during your illness. Use it for protection and also as an immune boost afterwards and you are likely to ward off a lot of colds and flu in the future.

Organic astragalus is increasingly available in herb stores dried and shredded. In Chinese pharmacies and Asian markets dried astragalus root looks like ice-lolly sticks. It is cheap and simple to prepare and it makes a mild, sweet tea. Look for sticks which are long and thick, firm yet bendable with a few striations. They should have a sweet taste when you chew on them.

One of the best ways in the world to take tonic and strengthening herbs is as foods. To the right is one of my favourite recipes for long cold winters. It uses potent immune strengthening herbs, in particular astralagus and burdock roots.

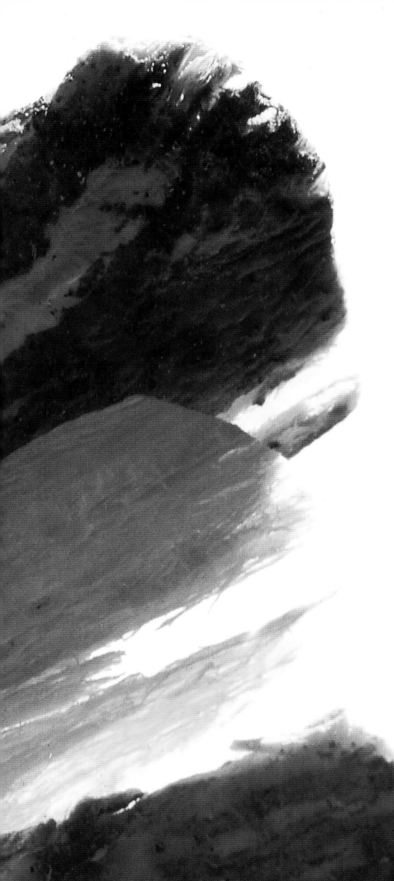

astragalus tea

- 6 sticks astragalus
- 3 pieces liquorice root sticks
- 5 cm (2 in) fresh ginger, peeled and sliced thinly
- 1½ litres (2½ pints) cold water

I make enough astragalus tea for four cups at a time – enough for a whole day. This recipe can make a sweet chilled drink but I prefer to reheat mine and drink it warm. Put the astragalus, liquorice root sticks and sliced ginger into a saucepan (not aluminium or non-stick). Pour the cold water over the herbs and bring the mixture to the boil. Reduce the heat and simmer for 20 minutes. Take it off the heat and allow to stand for 10 minutes. Strain and keep in the fridge.

herb tonic soup

- ½ cup brown rice or pearl barley
- 25 g (1 oz) dried, sliced astragalus root
- 25 g (1 oz) dried, sliced burdock root
- ginger root, finely chopped
- pinch of salt
- 1 large onion, diced
- 2 carrots, diced
- ½ red or green pepper, diced
- parsley, chopped
- garlic

Make 2 pints of vegetable stock from leftover vegetables or use Marigold Swiss Vegetable Bouillon Powder in a large pan. Add the rice or barley, astragalus, burdock, ginger (to taste) and salt and let the soup simmer for 1 hour. In a little olive oil quickly fry the diced onion, carrot and red or green pepper and add to the simmering stock mixture and simmer for another 30 minutes. Just before serving, remove the astragalus and add as good a handful of chopped crushed raw garlic as you can manage!

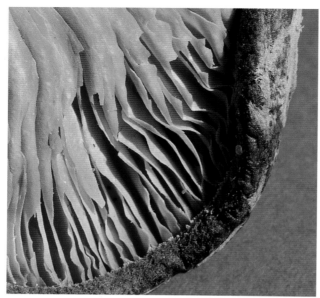

▲ shiitake mushroom   ► echinacea

listen to the japanese

Shiitaki and maitaki mushrooms not only taste delicious, they also contain excellent immune strengthening compounds, among them the compound lentinan. This phytochemical helps lower elevated cholesterol. It also boasts anti-ageing and anti-tumour properties. You can take shiitaki and maitaki mushrooms in capsules or as extracts but I prefer eating the mushrooms themselves. I soak the dried mushrooms and put them in soups and stews and stir-fries.

gifts from the sea

Kelp is a catch-all word. It covers a wide variety of sea plants from bladderwrack (*Fucus vesiculosus*) to the big leafed brown algae laminaria. Sea plants are perfect for restoring minerals and trace elements – and therefore strength and resilience – to a person who has lived for years on convenience foods depleted of them. Seaweeds are also rich in iodine, which helps keep your thyroid healthy.

Use these sea plants in your soups and salads – indeed, in all your savoury recipes, or eat them on their own. Sheets of nori are delicious toasted for 10 seconds under a grill.

purple potency

The lovely echinacea flower is the best known antiviral plant. As a result, sadly, it has also become one of the most expensive. Extracts of echinacea root behave like interferon – your body's own internal virus fighter. Echinacea contains at least three plant chemicals that have immune strengthening antiviral activities – echinaceine, chicoric acid and caffeic acid. As yet, nobody is sure if this is what gives the plant its power. What is known for sure is that echinacea increases your body's levels of an important immune activator known as properdin, which despatches white blood cells to do battle with invaders. I am sure it is the combined synergy of the plant that does the trick.

Purple cone flower or Black Sampson is a plant native to the prairies of North America with hard-to-beat properties to stimulate the immune system, heal wounds, enhance skin, counter infection and calm inflammation. The Sioux used it for snake bites, blood poisoning and wound healing. Until the twentieth century its roots and rhizomes were primary agents for the treatment of fever and infections from flu and colds to serious conditions like typhoid, meningitis, malaria, diphtheria, boils and abscesses.

When drugs came into being in a big way the beautiful echinacea plant was almost forgotten – except in Germany. There researchers began to quantify its effects on the body, discovering that it has properties equal to and often greater than most antibiotics to prevent and heal infection. It offers cortisone-like anti-inflammatory activity, interferon-like activity to heighten immunity and an ability to stimulate T-cells – important mediators in the body's immune system.

Used throughout periods of stress echinacea, which contains two polysaccharides called inulin and echinaceine, reinforces the body's defence mechanisms. This makes it easy to ward off colds and flu as well as fungal infections. The body is continually detoxified and its vital powers to resist illness are strengthened. The immunostimulatory activities of echinacea make it a bold ally in fighting off viral or bacterial infections including boils, abscesses and carbuncles as well as healing wounds.

Echinacea can even help slow down the rate at which the body and skin age. This property comes in part as a result of its ability to prevent the breakdown of one of the body's primary defence mechanisms – the so-called H-system of hyaluronic acid. Hyaluronic acid is the intercellular cement that forms a barrier against infection and helps keep skin strong, resilient and youthful. As the body ages, an enzyme attacks the hyaluronic acid so it loses its viscosity and changes from a firm jelly to a thin, watery fluid. Echinacea blocks the enzyme's effects. This inhibits the spread of infection and maintains good collagen and elastin in the skin, keeping skin looking young.

daily daisy

Echinacea is to plants what vitamin C is to vitamins – everyone is taking it and these days you can hardly find a remedy that doesn't contain it. You can use capsules of the ground herb – 1 to 4 capsules three to four times a day depending on whether it is being used as a prophylactic or treatment for illness. Or if you prefer, take the plant tincture as ½ to 1 teaspoon in a little water two or three times a day for prevention, or several times a day as treatment – up to 2 teaspoons an hour for a day or two at the onset of illness.

echinacea on the rocks

Next time you reach for a highball, ask yourself if that is what you really want. You might like to try a herbal tincture instead. I often drink them when I have a particular need – just the way you would a highball mixed with a little water over rocks. Throughout the Middle Ages it was the monks who prepared alcohol-based liquids from plants and flowers for healing. They knew all the secrets: that tincture of St John's wort helps banish melancholia; that tincture of passionflower is great as a night cap; that tincture of ginger can calm a troubled stomach. One of my favourite herbal highballs is tincture of echinacea, either *Echinacea angustifolia* or *Echinacea purpurea*, on the rocks. I use it daily when I am working (or playing) too hard and too long and want to make sure my immune system doesn't let me down.

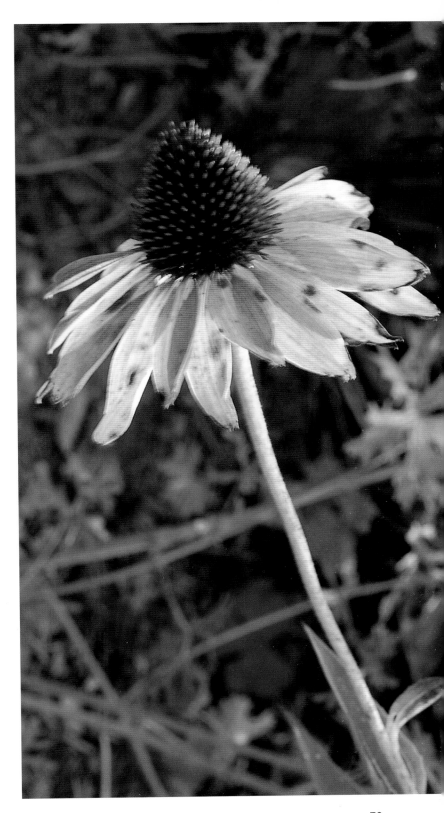

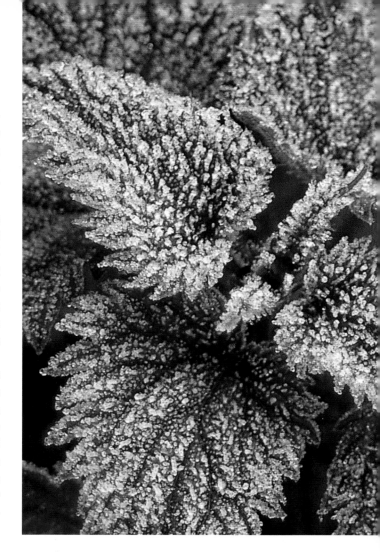

put a sting in your tail

Nettle (*Urtica dioica*) is the one plant everybody recognizes – and reviles. It's often the first plant we learn to identify as children. You don't quickly forget the pain that comes with grabbing a handful of stinging nettle. You soon learn too that the quickest way to relieve your misery is to pick a dock leaf and rub it on the sting.

It is this early lesson to keep well away from nettle that makes many people wary of using it as a herbal remedy. Don't hesitate. Nettle is a wonderful strengthening tonic for the blood – great for mild anaemia. It also strengthens the stomach against digestive disturbances. And nothing stems heavy bleeding like stinging nettle. Doctors have used it for at least two centuries to keep wounded soldiers from bleeding to death. Nettle's ability to sting is negated by drying or cooking.

Nettle is a plant that strengthens the liver, cleanses the blood and may even help you lose resistant excess fat from your body at the same time. Nettle loves rich soil and as a result is rich in vitamin C, calcium, magnesium, iron and potassium. This richness makes it a good tonic for the whole system drunk as a tea three times a day. Gather your nettle leaves in early summer before the plant flowers. Don't try to use nettle that has already flowered because it can be so strong by then that it irritates rather than helps.

nettle soup

► *1½ litres (3 pints) vegetable boillon or broth*
► *3 potatoes, diced in their skins*
► *1 medium-sized onion, chopped*
► *6 cloves garlic*
► *several handfuls fresh nettles*
► *powdered kelp*

Bring the vegetable bouillon or broth to the boil in a large saucepan and then add the potatoes, onion and garlic and boil for 15 minutes. Toss several handfuls of the fresh nettles into the soup and simmer for another 10 minutes. Remove from the heat and pour into a food processor or blender to liquidize. Add powdered kelp to taste.

nettle tea

► *1 litre (2½ pints) water*
► *handful nettle leaves*

Bring the water to the boil. Take it off the stove and toss in a large handful of the nettle leaves, freshly chopped. Cover the mixture and allow it to steep for an hour. Strain and chill.

▲ nettle

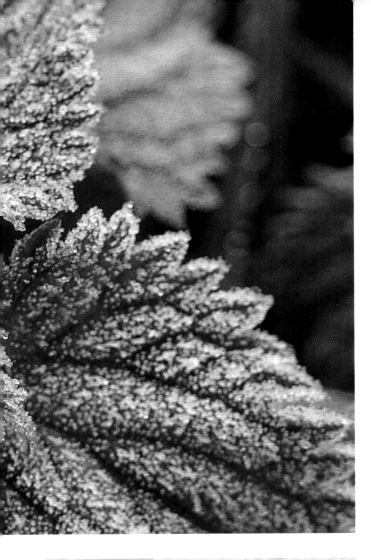

Each year you hear about some new strain of flu set to disrupt our lives and make the winter months miserable. But why use the latest flu vaccine when herbs work better and are safer? After all, we know little about the long-term consequences of immunization. The success of the flu vaccine depends on the success of the manufacturers in deciding which virus is going to cause the most cases this year. The elderly, people with heart or lung disease and those whose immune systems have been compromized by diseases such as AIDS and cancer, may benefit from the flu vaccine simply because their risk of dying from complications is greater than a healthy person's. However, there are risks. Michael Carlston MD at the University of California says, 'The vaccine itself is a stress on the body and could potentially have unwanted effects on the immune system.' I never use them. Instead, I prefer using preventative herb treatments to keep me from being laid low by minor illnesses whether caused by bacteria or viruses.

If you are generally healthy yet lead a stressful lifestyle, the occasional cold is likely to be nothing more than your body's way of getting rest and clearing out wastes. But when you find yourself spending most of the winter with your nose in a handkerchief then it is time to look seriously at prevention. There are many plant friends that help protect you from colds and flu. Viruses cannot replicate themselves without entering the cells and altering their function. If you can stop the virus invading your cells, you will stop flu in its tracks.

go for C

It may sound excessive to take 4 g of vitamin C a day, but if you are under the weather or your immune system needs a boost, you will soak up vitamin C like blotting paper. It's worth remembering that we don't make our own vitamin C like other animals. If we were goats, we would be making at least 5 g of vitamin C a day for ourselves. The body flushes out any vitamin C it doesn't need. If you find your bowels are loose, reduce the amount you are taking. Look for a supplement that has bioflavonoids in it as well. Take 1-2 g of vitamin C twice a day with meals.

At the first sign of a cold:

◆ Take a dropperful of tincture of echinacea in water, and repeat the dose every hour.
◆ Pour boiling water into a bowl and add a few drops of tea tree or manuka oil, eucalyptus and peppermint oil. Inhale the steam, allowing the antibacterial properties of the tea tree to ward off the cold and the peppermint and eucalyptus to prevent congestion.
◆ Increase your intake of vitamin C.
◆ Don't try to go to work as you will simply be spreading your illness around.
◆ Drink lots of fluids, but not milk as it can irritate the immune system.
◆ If respiratory problems do not improve quickly, consult your doctor.

science meets nature

Every so often you come upon a perfect marriage of nature and science in the service of man. Olive leaf extract is just such a one. It is a major natural antibacterial and antiviral herb, capable of countering even the so-called superbugs such as resistant strains of *Staphylococcus aureus*. These are bacterial beasties which even the best antibiotics won't dent.

The awareness that olive leaves contain immune strengthening phytochemicals including the antiviral aleuropein is not new. But only recently have we been able to make full use of its power. The problem has been that the processing of olive leaves with heat, or using the wrong kind of leaves from the wrong kind of trees – even having the leaves broken – meant that the protective potency of the plant was destroyed. Olive leaf extract only works on the human body when it chemically binds with blood serum. Scientists have worked with this challenge for several years and recently they have discovered a method of processing olive leaves that preserves their health benefits. It comes to us in the form of a highly concentrated powdered olive leaf extract. You can buy it in bulk or in capsules. You can even find olive leaf extract in concentrated liquid form. I prefer the capsules. It takes 1 litre (2½ pints) of ordinary liquid extract to produce even one capsule of this quite amazing stuff.

flu – a thing of the past

The new olive leaf extract can be used to strengthen the whole of you against illness when used in a preventative way by taking a couple of capsules a day. Taking it in this way reduces your risk of contracting flu strains types A, B and C. But olive leaf extract is not cheap and you need to make sure that you buy a good product from a reliable source (see Resources). The same olive leaf extract is also useful if you come down with flu. And it counters other viruses responsible for lower respiratory tract

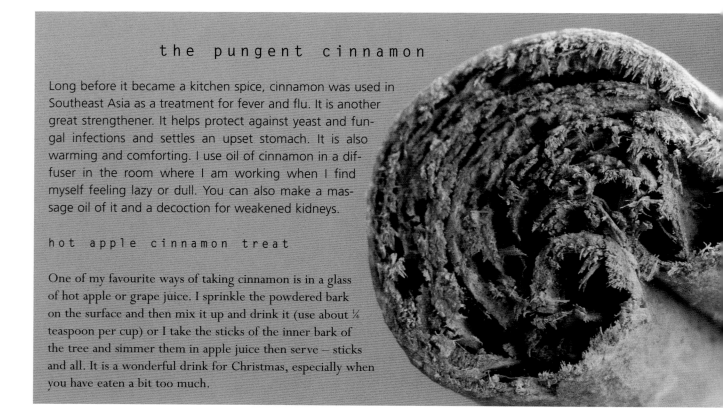

the pungent cinnamon

Long before it became a kitchen spice, cinnamon was used in Southeast Asia as a treatment for fever and flu. It is another great strengthener. It helps protect against yeast and fungal infections and settles an upset stomach. It is also warming and comforting. I use oil of cinnamon in a diffuser in the room where I am working when I find myself feeling lazy or dull. You can also make a massage oil of it and a decoction for weakened kidneys.

hot apple cinnamon treat

One of my favourite ways of taking cinnamon is in a glass of hot apple or grape juice. I sprinkle the powdered bark on the surface and then mix it up and drink it (use about ¼ teaspoon per cup) or I take the sticks of the inner bark of the tree and simmer them in apple juice then serve – sticks and all. It is a wonderful drink for Christmas, especially when you have eaten a bit too much.

infections, helping to clear symptoms – from fever, cough and sore throat to pains, chills and general malaise. It is even effective against the common cold.

The new olive leaf extract has been used to defeat the virulent herpes simplex virus type 2 (HSV-2) passed through sexual contact. Genital herpes is considered virtually impossible to get rid of. It is a condition that first erupts about a week after being exposed to a partner who is infected. Once the virus is established in your body, it sets up a latent infection of the sacral sensory nerve ganglia from where it continues to reinfect the genitals, bringing a lot of pain to people who have been unfortunate enough to pick it up.

Finally, olive leaf extract also works against yeasts such as candida albicans, fungal infections, parasites – both protozoa and helminthic worms – and retroviruses. And it is a godsend in helping to eliminate chronic fatigue syndrome as well as in combating the rhinovirus – probably the most common cause of the common cold. I keep a bottle of olive leaf extract in my herbal medicine chest and carry another with me wherever I travel. You simply can't get any better than this when it comes to strengthening.

elderberry protection

Elderberries make an excellent tea. If you are one of those people who seem only to recover from one illness when another hits, these wonderful berries can help break the chain and give you a chance to recover completely. They will also greatly shorten the length of any time you are ill. The way they work against flu is fascinating: the flu virus breaks into healthy cells by piercing them with spikes on its surface. In some way that is not yet completely understood, elderberry appears to make these spikes useless, defeating the virus before it can do any damage. Take ½ to 1 teaspoon of elderberry tincture in a little water every 4 hours as soon as you feel the first symptoms. Continue to do this for three days to make sure you have thoroughly massacred the virus.

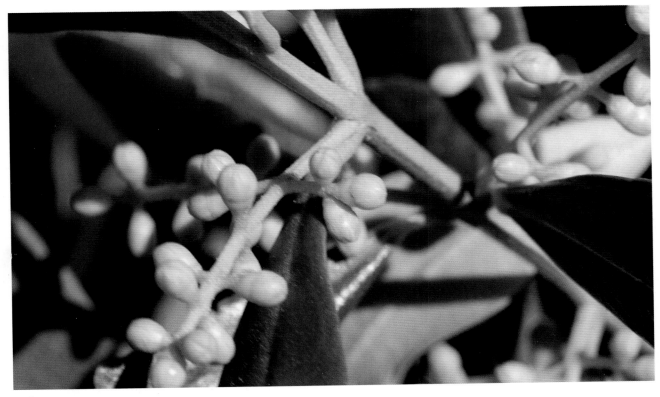

▲ olive

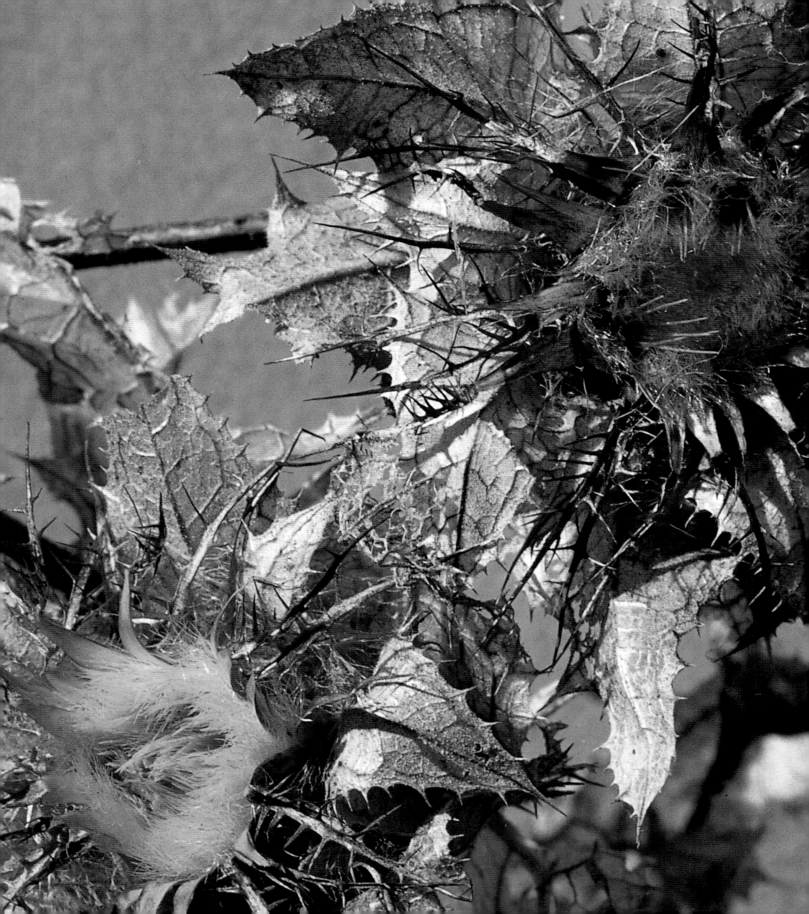

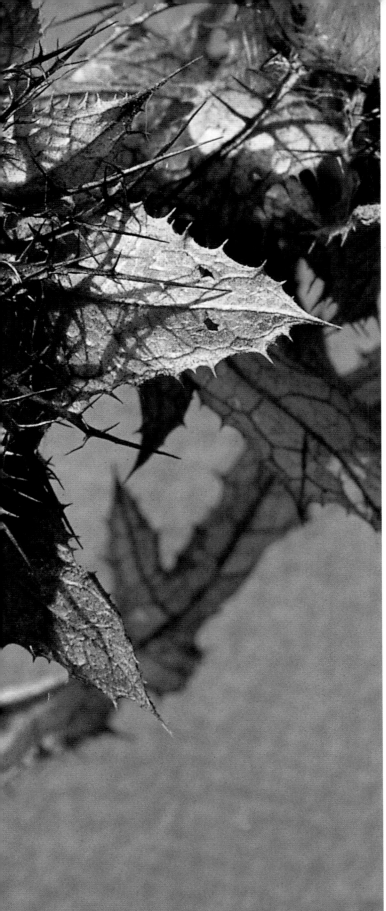

sanctifying 4

The most wondrous gift herbs ever bring me is not their dazzling power to heal and strengthen, but their magnificent beauty. I am moved to the very core whenever I take time to notice the way a plant looks and smells, when I sense the inexorable persistence of its growing, and the willingness it has to grace our lives with its delicate splendour. When you are aware of a plant's beauty at every level, even the most commonplace interaction with it becomes something sacred.

◄ blessed thistle

scented space

Fill your home with the beauty of herbs, grow plants in your kitchen and your bedroom ...

Place herbs on your desk or where you work. Burn sage and copal gold, lavender and natural incense to sanctify the environment. Make gifts for friends. Use herbs to care for your pets, to cleanse the space in which you live and work. This helps remind us of who we really are and what is fundamentally important in the de-sacralized environment in which we spend most of our life. For instance, I fill my bedroom with lilies. They are my favourite flowers. Over the years, I have come to know lilies very well. I know that they are most fragrant between two and three in the morning. The beauty of their fragrance is so intense that it often awakens me. Sometimes when this happens it seems to me that these flowers – so generous with their gifts – are calling to me, asking me to celebrate their wondrous beauty.

The word perfume comes from the Latin *per fumum* meaning 'through the smoke'. The original way in which fragrance was used in human life was to create a union of divine and mundane reality not only in the lives of priests but of ordinary people. Our sense of smell plays a powerful role in rituals. And ritual is one of the means by which we create the bridges between the transcendent and the day-to-day. Say a prayer before you eat. The very act of eating a meal takes on a magic act that nourishes not only your body but your soul as well.

scent of the devil

The ancient Egyptians believed that incense was the sweat of gods that had fallen to earth. We associate saints with beautiful fragrances and devils and evil spirits with foul smells. I remember once visiting an onsen in the mountains of Japan – a place of healing where hot, sulphurous water pours forth from natural underground wells. I walked down endless corridors before reaching the sulphur pool, which was enclosed to make it possible for people to use it even during the icy win-

ter months. I was alone in the small room. The pool sides were encrusted with yellow growths of sulphur and its sulphurous steam filled the room. As I climbed naked into the steaming water, I felt afraid. That is how deeply ingrained our sense of uneasiness can be when faced with the overwhelming smell of sulphur that our culture and ancestors associated with the Devil.

In Japanese legends incense is believed to attract goblins – jiki-ko-ti – and negative spirits such as the souls of men who during their lives had not honoured truth and beauty. As a result they were doomed to be attracted to incense smoke and wafted away on it. Religious rituals all over the world use fragrant burning plants to cleanse space, to sanctify and communicate with their deities. We first inherited the Christian practice of burning incense in churches from the Hebrews and Romans. Then in the sixteenth and seventeenth centuries incense began to grace the homes of the wealthy. Artisans of the time began to fashion incense not only into cones but into candles, tablets, birds and animals. They were used to sweeten the air and replace the fetid smells in their lives.

make it sacred

When you move into a new home or you feel a need to cleanse and make sacred any space – bedroom, kitchen, workroom or whole house – do it with the traditional sacred plants: sage, copal, sweetgrass or even dried lavender, thyme and rosemary.

I cut my herb plants back three or four times a year. They love it. It makes them grow stronger and bushier. I then take the cuttings and tie them in small bunches with brightly coloured ribbons and hang them from my kitchen ceiling to dry. Once dry I use them for potpourris, sachets and, of course, sanctifying space with their smoke.

sanctifying space

Take a bunch of dried herbs and light them over an open metal biscuit tin to catch the sparks so they don't reach the floor. I use a long, rectangular tin that once held a bottle of malt whisky for this. I know other people who use baking trays and turkey tins. When the herbs begin to smoke, walk around the space to be sanctified, lifting up the burning plants with the tin beneath them. All the while ask with your heart and mind that the room be cleansed and dedicated to whatever purpose you intend for it. This could be to make a joyous, harmonious space, a place in which creativity flourishes, or a space for meditation or sleep or prayer or making love. It is your intention coupled with the cleansing abilities of the burning plants that makes it happen.

When cleansing and dedicating a room, a house, an office, or any other space, ensure that you offer up the smoke to all the corners of the room and to the six directions – north, south, east, west, above and below. When you have finished thank the plants for their help.

go for the best

I use incense a lot. I like Japanese incense best because it is the finest and subtlest in the world. So much of what you find on the market is poor quality – made from sickly chemical fragrances rather than natural plant oils and resins. But the best Japanese incense can be hard to come by unless you go to Japan. So I have taken to making my own and have explored the best plants to burn either singly – as in the case of dried sage, cedar or sweetgrass – or mixed together and placed on top of a smouldering piece of charcoal (see box below).

Use incense for pleasure or to sanctify space. Burn incense by your bed, at the entrance to your house or on

my favourite plants for burning

Cedar: Native Americans burn cedar while praying so that their hopes and dreams, wishes and longings can rise on the smoke to the Creator. Cedar smoke, they say, builds a bridge between heaven and earth. Incense cedar purifies a room, banishes nightmares and uplifts the human spirit. It drives out negative energy and attracts good energies. It is also burned in sweat lodges to clear 'heavy emotional energies'.

Copal: Used by the Mayan Indians, copal is the pitch from their sacred tree. They burned it during divination ceremonies to nourish the gods. Copal is pregnant with spiritual power. The Mayan and Aztec royal families had their teeth filled with copal to give their speech divine clarity. Scientific researchers examining copal discovered that the smoke from it heightens immunity and strengthens the body. This is my very favourite of all the plant substances for burning. Copal smoke seems to cut through all the mental rubbish that so often clutters my mind, refilling it with clarity, energy and creativity. I use it all the time when I am beginning a day's writing.

Desert sage: This dried plant is used to strew the floor of holy places and also sweat lodges. Wherever sage is present, negative forces cannot enter.

Juniper: Like cedar, the needles of juniper are also used to banish negative energy.

White sage: Sweet and crisp is the smoke from dried white sage leaf. It is used for cleansing and sanctifying people, objects and places. Sage is one of the herbs elders traditionally use to smudge a person wishing to be healed for they need to be cleared of negative thoughts and feelings before the healing can take place. White sage is also useful for getting rid of the negative aftermath of anger.

Yerba santa: Drive out negative influences in a place with yerba santa and make a protective boundary against their returning. It also creates a good atmosphere for any healing sanctuary. Yerba santa helps hidden weaknesses, untruths, fears and disease come to the surface to be eliminated.

your desk. I burn incense before I work each day. I light it to honour the space in which I live when I return home. Be sure to protect the surfaces on which you burn home-made incense for when you put it on fuming charcoal it can burn a hole through surfaces. To protect my furniture, I heat a little round block of charcoal (you can buy them in packets from health-food stores) over a candle until it is glowing and put it in a pot that stands on a square of wood. I then drop small pieces of cedar, copal or lavender flowers on to the charcoal where they smoulder and fill the room with fragrant smoke. The square of wood gets marked by the heat, and I take care not to touch the pot until it has cooled down.

natural incense

To make your own incense you will need some charcoal to make it burn and maybe a bit of saltpetre to keep it burning, some fragrant herbs and essential oils, and something to bind them together like gum arabic or gum tragacanth.

Use pure powdered charcoal: the kind they use in churches all over the world. It burns with virtually no smell and produces a glow that allows essential oils to volatize and the herbs to smoulder. You can get pure charcoal from a chemist, or anywhere that sells church supplies. Don't try to use the stuff you burn on your barbecue as this has an unpleasant, acrid smell.

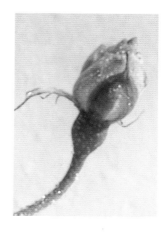

holy beads

I can't be sure, but I believe that 'rosaries' were once literally made out of strings of rose beads. They were certainly traditionally made of some sort of scented beads as the fragrance released as you handled them was meant to make

binding agents

▶*gum tragacanth*
▶ *2 tsp tragacanth powder*
▶ *300 ml (½ pint) warm water*

Dissolve the tragacanth powder in the warm water, continuing to stir until you have a consistency like wallpaper paste. Put it in a jar and give it a good shake to help break up any lumps. Keep your jar in a cool place, but not in the fridge, for three days, shaking it every day.

▶*gum arabic*
▶ *1 tbsp gum arabic*
▶ *2 tbsp boiling water*

Put the gum arabic into the boiling water and mix until you have a wallpaper paste consistency. Then put it into a bottle and shake to get rid of the lumps.

making incense

▶*14 tsp powdered charcoal*
▶ *½ tsp saltpetre*
▶ *3 tsp dried, powdered herbs*
▶ *1 tsp powdered resin*
▶ *1½ tsp essential oil*
▶*binding agent (see above)*

Grind the charcoal, saltpetre, herbs and resin to a fine powder in a mortar.
Mix the dry ingredients together. Add your essential oils and mix again. Add a little of the binding agent at a time until you have made a thick paste. Knead on a piece of oiled, greaseproof paper, and form into 2.5 cm (1 in) high cones or little round, flat pastilles. Dry them in a dark, airy place. (They will go mouldy if you put them in a box or don't allow the air to circulate around them freely.) When they are completely dry store them in a cool, dry place for when you need them.

its way to God and encourage Him to answer your prayers. Making rose beads is a labour of love – like an ongoing sacred offering. It was once carried out with reverence and much prayer.

collecting beauty

You will need a small mountain of rose petals – the more scented the better. Collect them when the dew has dried. The traditional method was to put the petals a little at a time into a mortar and grind them to a paste. In this day and age you can put them in a blender. Then you need to put the paste in a cast-iron saucepan. It is the reaction of the rose-petal paste with the iron that will make the beads black. Pour in just enough water (or even better, rose water) to cover the paste and gently heat it for about an hour. Don't let it boil. Allow it to cool then heat for another hour.

Put the paste back into the mortar and grind again. If your patience has run out and your paste is quite thick, you can try making the beads now. For a really top-class job, however, grind the paste a little every day for another week, or even two.

Now for the fun bit. Spread a little rose oil on your hands for extra fragrance and, taking a small amount of the rose-clay, roll it into a bead about twice the size of the bead you want to end up with. Push a large needle through the bead to make a hole (heat the needle if necessary) and string it on to fishing line or florist's wire. Repeat the process over and over again until you have used up all the rose-clay.

Then hang up the florist's wire or fishing line so the beads can dry. Turn them every day so they don't stick. In about two weeks they will have shrunk to half their original size and be ready for finishing.

Take a soft cloth and polish the beads until they look like old ebony. You can then string them on to a necklace in whatever way you like. When worn against the skin they will release the most beautiful captured scent of your roses.

rosemary incense

spicy Welsh incense

These two recipes are for you to experiment with. Soon you will be making up your own.

▶20 parts dried rosemary leaf powder
▶10 parts charcoal powder
▶4 parts benzoin powder
▶1 part saltpetre powder
▶5 parts essential oil of rosemary
▶5 parts essential oil of myrrh
▶Gum arabic as needed

▶12 parts charcoal powder
▶40 parts sandalwood powder
▶15 parts benzoin powder
▶3 parts saltpetre
▶3 parts cubeb powder
▶4 parts ground cinnamon
▶1 part myrrh powder
▶3 parts vanilla oil
▶5 parts lemon grass oil
2 parts ylang ylang oil
▶Gum arabic as needed

fragrant herbs to choose from

resins to add to your herbs

Use any essential oils you feel might go well with your chosen herbs and resins. Don't be afraid to experiment.

▶Angelica seeds
▶Bay leaves
▶Cinnamon
▶Cloves
▶Juniper leaves
▶Lavender flowers
▶Marjoram
▶Orris root
▶Rosemary leaves
▶Sandalwood
▶Star anise
▶Thyme leaves

▶Angelica resin
▶Balsam of Peru
▶Benzoin
▶Camphor
▶Frankincense
▶Myrrh
▶Terebinth

Go gently as resins can overwhelm the smell of everything else.

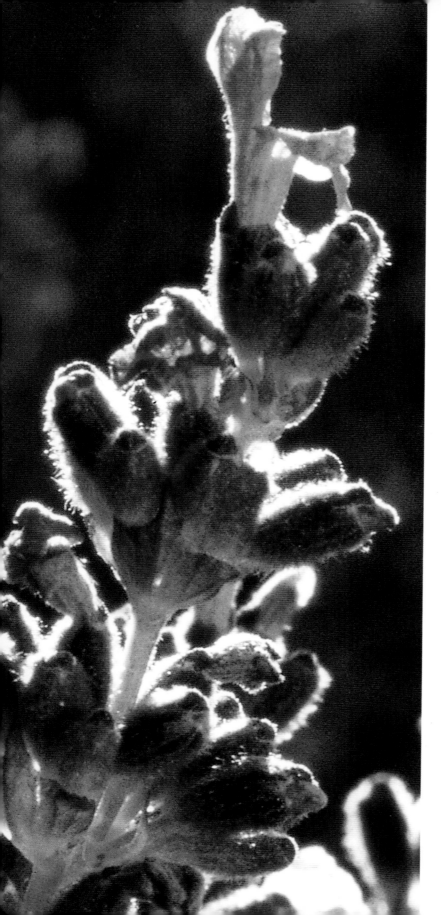

heaven scent

The value of essential oils ...

Humans have probably used herbs to make their homes beautiful and comfortable for a million years. The scent of herbs is as natural to us as spring rain breaking through sunshine. Both our ability to smell and our experience of intense emotions such as joy, fear, desire, or rage are governed by the limbic system – the brain's most primitive part. That is probably why even the slightest hint of a smell can be so emotionally evocative. When you smell something beautiful – or ugly – you are reacting to volatile molecules wafting their way to odour receptors behind the bridge of your nose. From there, nerve impulses are carried to the limbic system, the messages are interpreted and responses are sent by the hypothalamus to the rest of your body. Scent not only affects you emotionally but physically, psychologically and spiritually.

essential truths

Some of the most powerful message carriers are the essential oils of plants – the distilled essences of leaves, fruits, flowers, bark and roots. They are brimming with structural information – the complex energies of life itself. Each aromatic essence carries a different message to your body: vanilla and lavender, for instance, tell it to relax, while peppermint and rosemary encourage it to wake up. Some Japanese companies have capitalized on this. They pump essential oils like lemon through the air-conditioning of their offices to increase productivity in their workers. Whenever you become bored or drowsy, diffusing the right essential oil into the atmosphere can shift your energy on every level and revive you.

Essential oils can also help clarify mental states and balance emotions. Use them to help clear the fog from your brain after a hard day's work. Use them all over

◀ lavender

your home to intensify whatever atmosphere you've been trying to achieve with colour, textures and decoration. I use lemon verbena, hyssop and neroli when I am working and ylang ylang, lavender or vanilla in the bath to wind down at the end of the day.

There are all sorts of methods for enriching your room with the uplifting energy of essential oils. You can put them in an oil burner. Fill the saucer on the top with water before adding a few drops of your preferred oil (the water is important because burning these essences neat destroys much of their beauty and power). There are machines on the market which you plug in so an electric fan wafts the fragrance into the air without heating. A simple diffuser comes in the form of a ring which you place around a light bulb. The heat from the bulb evaporates any oil you drop on to it, diffusing it into the atmosphere. Or put 8-10 drops of essential oils on a small piece of cardboard or in a dish of warm water and leave it on a warm radiator or Aga stove.

A method I really like is to make a room spray by filling a spray bottle with water and adding 2 drops of washing-up liquid and 10 drops of my favourite essential oil. I not only use this throughout my home but I take a bottle of it wherever I travel so I can spray my hotel room. It makes me feel much more comfortable in a strange place. Here are my suggestions (see below) for using essential oils to enhance your environment.

summer bowls

I also fill my home with bowls of potpourri in winter. It is an offering I make to my house to remind it of the

living space	desired effect	essential oils
Living room	Calming	◆ Geranium: relieves anxiety ◆ Clary sage: clears the head after mental activity ◆ Vanilla: brings home comforts and childhood memories
Bedroom	Soothing	◆ Camomile: calms panic and helps with insomnia ◆ Ylang ylang or jasmine: ease depression and are aphrodisiac
Bathroom	Relaxing	◆ Lavender or vanilla: calm irritability ◆ Rosemary or pine: act as a tonic for the nerves
Office space	Energizing	◆ Basil: clears the mind and banishes indecision ◆ Cedarwood: clears the mind and heightens creativity ◆ Neroli: heightens mental functioning
Dining room	Entertaining	◆ Jasmine: helps counter shyness ◆ Sandalwood: opens the mind to new ideas
Kitchen	Uplifting	◆ Lily: restores energy ◆ Peppermint: lifts the spirits ◆ Coffee or cocoa: draws your guests into the kitchen and makes food taste better

colours and smells of the summer and a promise that it will come again. Many shop-bought potpourris smell sickly. Many are highly unnatural, full of artificially coloured petals, leaves and shavings and unpleasant phony smells. I much prefer the home-made variety full of herbs, leaves and flowers picked fresh and dried naturally. These summer gleanings make wonderful potpourri gifts – given in glass jars tied with ribbon, placed in a bowl you buy for pennies at a jumble or garage sale, or wrapped in a simple piece of muslin.

colour, scent and spice

There is no strict recipe for making potpourri. You can create your mixture from anything you like to look at, anything you like to smell, or whatever is in season when you begin. You will need some colour (leaves and petals), some scent (herbs), a little spice if you like (you can even raid the kitchen cupboards for this), a few drops of essential oil, and a fixative (see opposite). Try not to use anything that has been sprayed with pesticides or herbicides and don't use metal containers or utensils as the metal can react with the ingredients to alter the smell.

fresh pickings

Gather your herbs, flower heads, petals and buds at midday when any dew or rain has gone from them and they are dry. If you can, pick your flowers just after they have opened. This is when they have the highest concentration of essential oils. Spread them out on paper

potpourri ingredients

colour, texture

▶apple blossom	▶marigold	▶rose leaves
▶blackcurrant leaves	▶mock orange	▶rose petals
▶camomile	▶nasturtium	▶rose
▶delphinium	▶pansy	▶tansy
▶geranium leaves	▶pine cones	▶violets
▶goldenrod	▶rose buds	▶yarrow

spice

▶allspice	▶cloves	▶nutmeg
▶cardamom seeds	▶coriander seeds	▶star anise
▶cinnamon	▶ginger	

scent

▶angelica root	▶honeysuckle	▶myrrh
▶basil	▶hyssop	▶rosemary
▶bay	▶jasmine	▶sage
▶borage	▶lavender	▶sandalwood shavings
▶cedarwood shavings	▶lemon balm	▶stocks
	▶lemon verbena	
▶dried lemon peel	▶marjoram	▶thyme
▶dried orange peel	▶mint	▶vetivert root

a favourite recipe

To get you started here is one of my favourite recipes.

▶rose petals from about 3 dozen roses
▶handful each of petals from scented flowers such as lavender, rosemary, jasmine, mock orange
▶handful each of leaves from plants such as mint, bay, marjoram, geranium
▶few brightly coloured petals, such as delphiniums, marigolds
▶few pieces of angelica
▶little dried orange or lemon peel
▶100 g (4 oz) powdered orris root
▶25 g (1 oz) coriander seed
▶25 g (1 oz) grated nutmeg
▶25 g (1 oz) whole cloves
▶2 or 3 sticks of cinnamon
▶few drops of geranium essential oil
▶few drops of lavender essential oil

and make sure you throw out any leaves or petals that are going brown, as well as any green parts of roses. Removing leaves from stems and petals from flowers helps them to dry more quickly. Alternatively, tie flowers and leaves still on their stems in bunches and hang them somewhere warm to dry (my kitchen ceiling is always a good place). You might like to loosely tie a cheesecloth, muslin or paper bag around flowers like lavender to catch the flower heads that would otherwise drop all over the floor. (Remember to discard the centres of marigolds if you are going to use them for medicinal purposes.)

Dry your leaves and petals on the paper in a warm airy place, turning them frequently. If you have a drying screen or mesh, your mixture will dry even more quickly and preserve more of the essential oils. Orange and lemon peel will dry very easily. Simply remove as much of the fruit and pith as you can, break, grate or shave the skin into small pieces and leave until it's brittle.

Check your drying ingredients every day so that you don't risk losing them to mould. Once they are thoroughly dry, store them in airtight containers. If you conscientiously gather herbs and flowers throughout the spring and summer, you will have a wonderful array to play with by the autumn. Store the airtight containers all in a dark place, to preserve as much of the plants' colours as possible, until you are ready to use them.

spice it up

When you are ready to make your potpourri, see what spices you have in your kitchen cupboards. Spices, especially beautifully shaped ones like star anise, look wonderful scattered through any potpourri. Remember to freshly grind a little of each spice you use to add to the potpourri with the whole spices to make full use of their aroma.

Mix your herbs, leaves, flowers and spices of choice and put into an airtight container. It is at this point that you can decide whether you would like to add a little extra something to your mix by including essential oils. Two of my favourites for potpourri are geranium and lavender. Use essential oils sparingly as they can completely overwhelm any other scent. Add them drop by smallest drop at a time.

fix it

Using a fixative preserves the fragrance of your potpourri by slowing down the evaporation of essential oils. I use orris root – the powdered root of the Florentine iris. It has been known to cause allergic reactions in some people, so if you find you have a problem with it, try dried ground rosemary leaves, or dried ground vetivert root instead. I buy my orris root by the bag from my local health food store. You will need about a tablespoon of fixative to 1 litre (2 pints) of potpourri. Add it to your mixture and close the lid of your air-tight jar.

You will want to leave the potpourri for four to six weeks to allow the fragrances to blend. Give the jar a shake once a week and check it to see if the mixture is neither too wet nor too dry. If you think it is too wet, add a little extra orris root powder. If too dry, then add a little ordinary salt.

When your potpourri is ready, pour some of it into bowls around the house. Store the remainder sealed in a jar in a cool dark place. It should keep well so you can use it when and where you like later.

be professional

Whenever you make your own potpourri, take time to make a note of the ingredients and quantities you use. In this way you can re-create something you particularly liked. Believe me, you'll never manage it again if you don't write it down! As you become more experienced you might like to try putting together your potpourris the way 'noses' create perfume. Choose a main scent, which will be the bulk of the herbs you use. Then carefully consider which spices, woods and essential oils go well with that base scent.

scented bowl

If I don't have any potpourri and want to make a scented bowl for a room, perhaps for an unexpected guest, I tend to use whatever comes to hand. One of my favourites is to fill a small white bowl with dried white beans, which are so beautiful to look at. Then I simply add a few drops of essential oil and mix it in. Try using dried beans, grains, pebbles or small wooden balls.

bags of herbs

One of the things that makes a herb-loving house so special is the way herbs creep into every nook and cranny ...

They make the ordinary into something beautiful. Linen drawers strewn with herb sachets are a joy to open. Herb bags freshen wardrobes, enliven drawers and scent notepaper. Put them in the corners of cupboards and drawers to be used by guests. You can even tuck them among their pillows and make your guests feel like they have come home. Slip herb sachets down the back of the cushions on your sofa and you will be surrounded by the most delightful fragrance every time you sit down to relax.

A herb sachet is nothing more than a small fabric bag filled with perfumed dried herbs – in fact a potpourri which has been crumbled, sometimes even ground, so that the dried herbs fit into the sachet. You can use some of your own potpourri (see pages 91-3) and grind it in a mortar, or even in a coffee grinder, if you can't break it up with your fingers. Or you can dry other herb mixtures specifically for sachets. Make sure the herbs you use are absolutely dry. You don't want a mouldy old bag in among your underwear.

do-it-yourself

You can make your bags out of any material you like, but I think natural fabrics work far better than synthetics. Fabrics with a tight weave will hold the powdered herbs better than a loose-weave fabric – linen and silk are perfect. I have a passion for linen bedclothes. I like to think that linen sachets are the proper way to look after my sheets, so I make my herb sachets from old linen pillow cases. What size and shape you make them is entirely up to you. Traditionally, sachets for drawers were 5-7.5 cm (2-3 in) square. They were oblong for linen cupboards. You can make them large, tiny, heart-shaped or round, whatever takes your fancy. How you fill them depends on what you like and what you have to hand. Opposite are a few of my favourites.

▼ left to right: four basic herbs for sachets: lavender, lemon balm, mint and rose

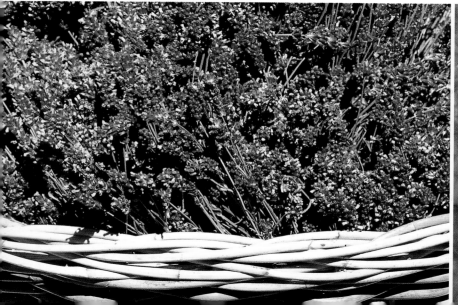

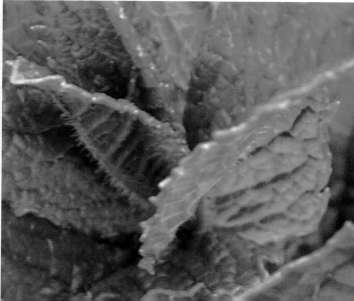

bags of gifts

Herb sachets make charming gifts, particularly if you decorate them yourself with embroidery silks or fabric paints. You can also slip them inside a needlepoint bag. Such gifts are not only for Great Aunt Maude, they make thoughtful presents for anyone who has just moved house and an unusual gift for men. You can put your sachet mix into anything made of fabric that will hold it. Use your imagination. Here are a few of my favourite gift ideas.

herb sachets

◆ **Lavender lovelies:** if, like me, you love lavender, simply fill your sachets with dried lavender flowers and sprinkle with a few drops of lavender essential oil before sewing up.

◆ **Summer sachets:** mix dried lavender flowers with dried peppermint leaves.

◆ **Mint madness:** collect leaves from as many different types of mint as you can find – spearmint, peppermint, apple mint, pineapple mint, ginger mint – dry them, grind them and put them into sachets for sock drawers.

◆ **Sentimental rose:** use rose petals collected from old-fashioned, highly scented flowers like musk roses. Be particularly careful that your petals are properly dried. Roses especially are prone to going mouldy. You can always add a few drops of rose essential oil, if you can find some that is natural and doesn't cost an arm and a leg – pure oil of rose is one of the most expensive.

herb gifts for men

◆ **Tie refreshers:** men's neck ties are hollow. If you tie a knot so the tie looks like it has just been loosened and taken off you can pour some sachet mixture into the wide end and sew it up. Men tend to prefer spicy scents to flowery ones, such as thyme, nutmeg and clove; lemon balm and cardamom or a selection of mint leaves. Hang it from a tie rack (but just make sure he doesn't mistake the sachet for a tie and try to wear it).

◆ **Car maintenance:** rather than buying an air freshener for the car, try filling a pair of driving gloves with sachet mix, sew them shut and leave them in the glove compartment. This is a real bonus on hot days when cars can smell and feel very stale.

◆ **Shoe fresheners:** put your sachet mix into a triangular bag, or even a pair of cotton socks and sew them up. You can then slip your sachets into pairs of shoes to protect those you don't often wear, and to freshen those you wear to work each day. They will even sweeten a teenager's old trainers.

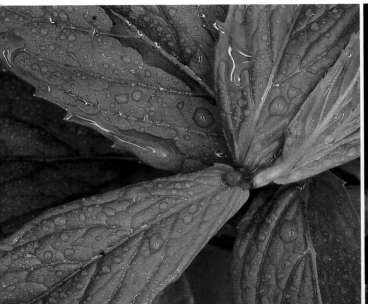
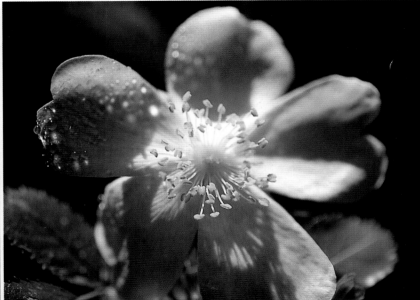

home is where the herbs are

Many commercial household cleaning products are fragranced with herbal smells – most of them, alas, artificial ...

This is not only because herbs have a long-lasting scent but because market research shows that if we smell a strong, aromatic herb in our washing-up liquid or disinfectant we automatically assume that it is going to do a good job. It's all to do with the associations we have with these smells. For centuries, herbs have been used in the home to ward off insects, keep illness at bay and generally make our living spaces pleasant, perfumed and comfortable places to be. Call it race memory if you like, but I think that we all associate the fragrance of herbs with cleanliness, homeliness and good housekeeping.

The problem with many of the cleaning products on our supermarket shelves is that they combine some rather nasty ingredients with a herbal fragrance. For instance, you may find the chemical NAT, listed as carcinogenic by the US National Cancer Institute, or compounds that can cause respiratory failure such as sodium nitrate; not to mention naphtha, which can seriously upset the central nervous system. I love the smell of herbs in my house but prefer to use products that are as clean as they smell, such as those given below and overleaf. Clean your house with pure herbal products and you will sanctify your home at the same time.

furniture polish

▶ *100 g (4 oz) beeswax*
▶ *300 ml (1 pint) turpentine*
▶ *essential oil*

Grate the beeswax into the turpentine. The beeswax needs to dissolve into the turpentine and it will do this naturally over a period of several days, but you can short-cut the process by putting the mixture into a double boiler on the stove and gently heating it until the wax melts. (Be very, very careful if you decide to use this method, however, as turpentine can easily catch fire.) Add a few drops of your chosen essential oil and stir into the mixture. My favourite oils for this are pine, lavender, thyme or rosemary. Pour the polish into a tin or jar and allow to set. Apply to furniture with a soft cloth. Let it dry and buff gently to create a shine you can see your face in. Your grandmother would be proud of you!

room spray

▶ *600 ml (1 pint) spray bottle*
▶ *essential oil*
▶ *washing-up liquid*

You can also make the most delicious room sprays using your favourite essential oils and water. Fill a spray bottle with water and 10 drops of your essential oil. Add a couple of drops of washing-up liquid to help the oils mix with the water and shake the bottle well otherwise the oils might clog up the spray. Then spray liberally around your house – it will uplift your spirits as well as make your home smell wonderful.

rich and warm

Using herbal preparations instead of commercially prepared cleaning products will bring your home alive. I travel a great deal and one of the nicest things about coming home is opening the front door to be greeted with the warm smell of furniture polish. I choose beeswax and turpentine as a base for a luxurious furniture polish. It may sound like something your great-grandmother used with gusto to make the floor treacherously shiny, but it makes a luxurious, creamy polish that enriches and protects anything made of wood. Furniture, frames, ornaments – and even leather upholstery – love the stuff and drink it in. To this base I add a few drops of essential oil so that the polish subtly scents wherever it touches.

strong and fresh

These days, advertisers use more and more food-related health scares to play upon our fear of germs and sell us potentially dangerous antibacterial products which pollute the environment and cause allergies in sensitive people. It seems that every kitchen cloth or cleaning product on the supermarket shelves is impregnated with strong disinfectants to make your work surfaces as sterile as a laboratory. Personally, I wouldn't prepare my food anywhere near them.

Instead, you can make your own kitchen sprays using nothing more than water and essential oils. Rosemary, sage, tea tree, manuka and eucalyptus are all naturally antimicrobial – perfectly capable of dealing with any day-to-day germs that might be hanging around the chopping board or kitchen surfaces. They smell great as well.

natural housekeeping

Delving into old housekeeping books and traditional herbals can be fascinating. Did you know, for instance, that horsetail used to be used as a pot scourer? Women gathered it, tied it into bunches and rubbed them around saucepans to make them gleam. I have learned lots of tricks that make housekeeping itself a loving act.

kitchen spray

▶ *600 ml (1 pint) spray bottle*
▶ *600 ml (1 pint) distilled, filtered, or still mineral water*
▶ *essential oil*
▶ *washing-up liquid*

Fill the spray bottle with the distilled, filtered, or still mineral water. Then add 10 drops of an essential oil such as rosemary, sage, tea tree or eucalyptus and put in 2-3 drops of washing-up liquid to help the oils mix with the water and shake well. Spray over your kitchen work surfaces and wipe them with a clean cloth.

kitchen disinfectant

▶ *1 tsp isopropyl alcohol*
▶ *2.5 litres (4 pints) water*
▶ *antimicrobial essential oil*
▶ *washing-up liquid (optional)*

For heavier-duty cleaning jobs I use isopropyl alcohol (available from any chemist) mixed with water and essential oils. Mix the isopropyl alcohol into the water and then add 20-30 drops of antimicrobial essential oils such as rosemary, sage, tea tree or eucalyptus. If you find the oils float to the surface, add a couple of drops of washing-up liquid.

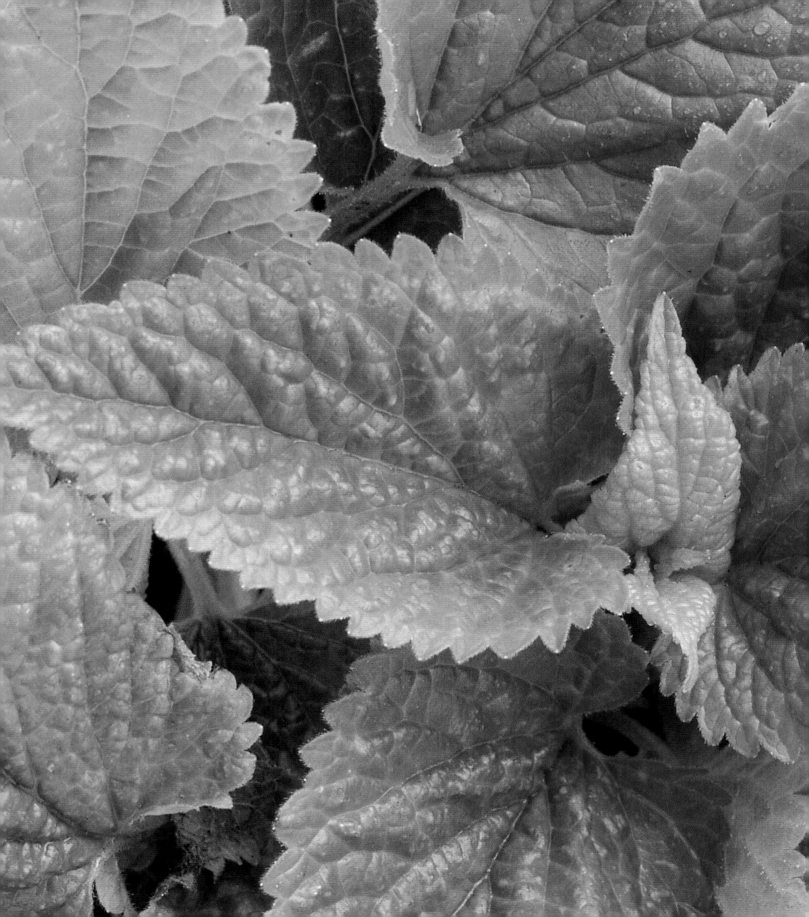

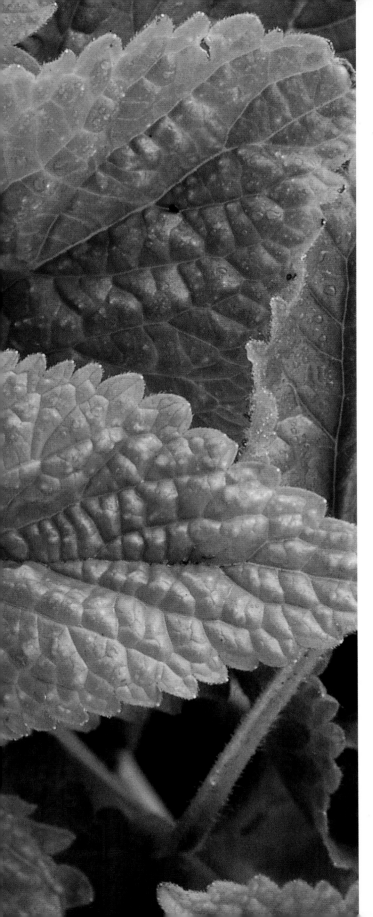

For example, I use a soft cloth soaked in lavender oil to remove mould from leather-bound books and prevent it from returning. I sprinkle a little of the oil on the bookshelf too, to help to keep mould away from other books – and because I love the smell. (Essential oils pack quite a punch so make sure not to use too much lavender oil or you can damage the delicate covers of old books and highly polished shelves – check by wiping a little lavender oil somewhere inconspicuous on the surface.)

Likewise, lemon balm leaves will give a wooden box a good shine and a delicious smell simply by rubbing the fresh leaves onto the wood and polishing with a soft cloth before it dries. You can polish pewter with fresh cabbage leaves, and clean silver with used lemon halves. Wipe the lemons over the silver, clean off with a warm damp cloth and give it a polish with a soft dry cloth.

metal cleaner

► *600 ml (1 pint) boiling water*
► *25-50 g (1-2 oz) horsetail*

Make a strong infusion of horsetail, pouring the water over the herb in a pan. Leave it to steep for a couple of hours. Then bring the infusion to the boil and simmer for 15 minutes. Strain into a large bowl and allow to cool. Immerse your metal objects into it and allow them to soak for 5 minutes. Take them out and let them dry, then buff them with a soft cloth.

lavender wash

► *25 g (1 oz) pure liquid soap*
► *½ cup washing soda*
► *6 drops essential oil of lavender*
► *½ cup borax (optional)*

Mix the pure liquid soap with the washing soda and then add the essential oil of lavender and mix. To make whites ultra-bright, add ½ cup borax (available from a chemist).

◄ lemon balm

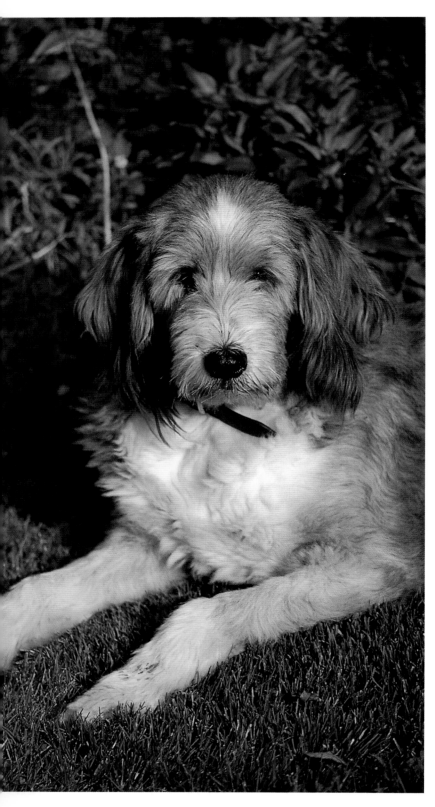

animal friends

We share our homes with
the best of creatures –
cats and dogs ...

Dogs have always been the great protectors of the home. Cats bring us a sense of mystery and enchantment. They never forget that they were worshipped in Ancient Egypt and that they honour your home with their sacred presence. Introduce herbs into the lives of your pets and they too will share in the cleansing, enhancing and sanctifying nature of plants. I have two Bearded Collies called Sunshine and Moonbeam, and two Burmese cats called Cappuccino and Carciofo (Italian for artichoke), who grace my life with love and affection, warmth – and fleas.

into the bath

My dogs are long-haired. I find I need to bathe them regularly, which helps discourage fleas. I use a mild tea tree shampoo and try to keep each dog in the water for

eucalyptus bath

► *4 tbsp dried eucalyptus leaves*
► *2 cups boiling water*
or
► *20 drops tea tree or eucalyptus oil*
► *600 ml (1 pint) water*

Put the dried eucalyptus leaves into a tea pot and cover with the boiling water. Leave the leaves to steep until cool and then strain. Alternatively, add the tea tree or eucalyptus oil to 600 ml (1 pint) of water in a spray bottle and then spray the mist all over your dog (but be sure to protect his or her eyes).

ten minutes to drown the fleas (not easy with Moonbeam!). Finally I give each dog a rinse with eucalyptus tea. Fleas really don't like the smell.

doggy pillows

For all their supposed toughness, dogs are comfort-loving creatures. I make flea-repelling herb pillows for my dogs' beds. I stuff an old pillow case with herbs and sew it up. I then slip this pillow inside another old pillow case as they get dirty quite quickly and I like to change them often. Try a mixture of pennyroyal, camomile flowers and dried rue. I always include pennyroyal in my doggy mix. Its Latin name is *Mentha pulegium*, *pulegium* coming from *pulex* (flea) in Latin. The name for the main chemical constituent in pennyroyal is pulegone. All of which proves that chemists do sometimes have a sense of humour.

When choosing herbs for your dog's pillow remember that their noses are much more sensitive than ours. You don't want to overwhelm them. There are times when this can be put to good use, however. Rubbing a little clove oil on the legs of furniture will discourage puppies from chewing them – but test out the clove oil somewhere inconspicuous to make sure it won't damage your furniture or you will be back to square one.

cat naps

It's not quite so easy with cats. Their saintly heritage makes them rather sensitive to strong smells, or anything that might dent their superior composure. Herbs like rue and pennyroyal, which repel fleas, also repel cats. I have found that some cats don't mind camomile so I put a little in my cats' pillows and mix in some catmint or valerian. Just about every cat I have ever met goes mad for valerian. To my nose it smells like the socks of soldiers who have been marching for two days. But, out of love for Chino and Choffie, as they are rather disrespectfully known, I make a few extra herb sachets with this mixture and scatter them in my linen cupboard, where they love to laze the day away.

As these pillows are smaller than dog pillows I suggest crumbling up the dried herbs. Use a mixture of camomile and catmint, or camomile and valerian. If you want to keep your cats off the furniture or from marking the curtains, use a strong room spray – it deters the animals but pleases the humans!

A note about catmint. There is an old saying that cats take little notice of the plants that grow from seeds sown straight into the garden. But when you raise the seed indoors, or buy some plants, and then transplant them into the garden the cats will literally love it to death. I have never tested this theory scientifically. I find that my cats chew the plant no matter how I grow it.

troubled ears

Ear mites are a very common problem in cats and irritating for them and you. Dribbling a few drops of garlic oil (peel a whole bulb of garlic, steep it for a week in 1.2 litres (2 pints) of olive oil, strain, bottle the oil and keep it in the fridge – and don't try to use essential oil of garlic, it's much too strong) into the ear twice a day will help enormously. Stop if your cat is made unhappy by the smell.

If, however, you have a young female being courted by the local tom cat and you don't want kittens, try putting a few drops of essential oil of garlic or squeeze a garlic capsule on the back of the female's neck. Her suitor is likely to be put right off his stride.

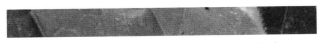

herbs for cats: to love and hate

▶ *600 ml (1 pint) spray bottle*
▶ *washing-up liquid*
▶ *½ tsp thyme essential oil*

Fill the spray bottle with water and add a couple of drops of washing-up liquid and the thyme essential oil. Shake the bottle well so the washing-up liquid helps the oil mix with the water. You can then spray this anywhere you want to keep cat-free – but test a small area first to make sure the room spray won't mark.

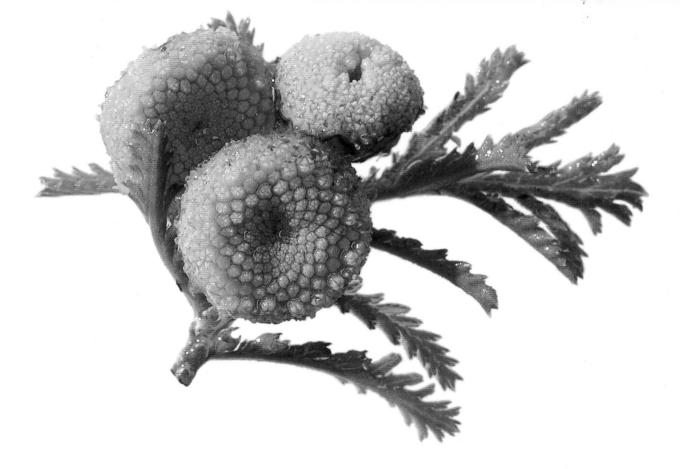

insect repellents

Everything in the universe has its proper place and function. Even maggots ...

Without them, decaying matter would not be broken down to make new life possible. It is only when something is out of place that things go wrong and a sense of the sacred is lost. After all, who wants maggots in their bed? In my view, the right place for insects is outside the house. Since humans began living indoors, herbs have been used to keep them there. In this age of toxic chemical sprays we can learn a lot from our ancestors about how to make our homes comfortable for humans yet uncomfortable for our companion pests. They used strewing herbs – sage and pennyroyal, tansy and lavender – and spread them on beaten earth floors. We can use the same herbs in dried bunches, in sachets and in sprays.

eliminate insects

In summer it can sometimes feel as though humans have no place in the kitchen. Flies perform intricate dances in the middle of the room, ants form queues to raid the shelves, and weevils quietly carouse in bags of flour and rice. I hate using chemical sprays anywhere. I would certainly never use them near food or in the vicinity of where I am going to prepare it. I rely on herbs.

Generally herbs repel insects, letting them know that they are not welcome in your home. For instance, I

▲tansy
► rue and southernwood

insect repellents for the home

Flies
- ◆ Make herb sachets (see page 95) from dried mint, cloves and eucalyptus and hang them near windows and doors.
- ◆ Hang fresh bunches of mint from window frames and doors.
- ◆ Grow pots of mint on window ledges and near to doors, inside and out.

Ants
- ◆ Hang a little bundle of fresh sage in cupboards where you keep food.
- ◆ Crush catnip or peppermint leaves on shelves where ants like to visit.
- ◆ Make herb sachets (see page 95) of dried pennyroyal, rue and tansy and tuck these into cupboards where you keep food.

Weevils
- ◆ Place a few dried bay leaves in flour, rice and pulses to keep weevils away.

Cockroaches
- ◆ Take essential oil of peppermint and 'paint' it where you know they live or wherever you have seen them.

Insects – in general
- ◆ Feverfew flowers are poisonous to most insects. Hang them in bunches from the ceiling or around windows. You can also make herb sachets of the dried, ground flowers and hang them in cupboards.
- ◆ If you get fed up with insects inviting themselves in through your windows, leave a peeled, halved onion on the window ledge.
- ◆ A lot of insects dislike sage. Hang it to dry in bunches around the house and from door and window frames. If you tie it with little ribbons in bunches it looks beautiful too.

moth-repellents
- ◆ Fill small sachets with cedarwood or southernwood shavings.
- ◆ Fill sachets with a mix of equal parts of rosemary, tansy and lavender.
- ◆ Fill sachets with a mix made of equal parts of dried mint, lavender and lemon verbena.
- ◆ Fill sachets with a mixture of equal parts of rosemary, vetivert and pennyroyal and add a few whole bay leaves.

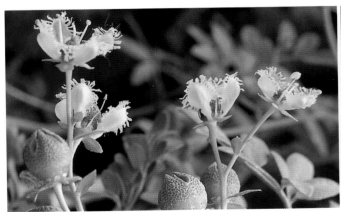
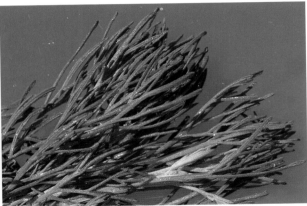

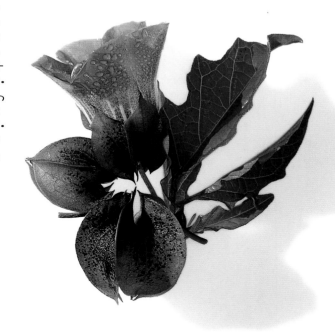

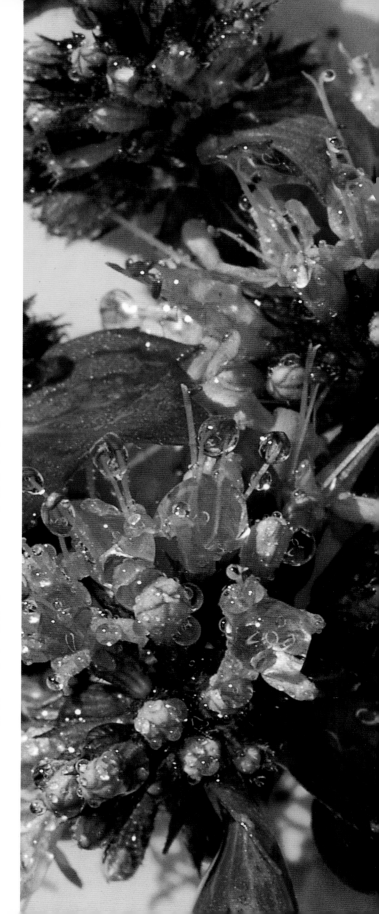

have discovered that ants dislike sage, catnip, pepper-mint, pennyroyal, rue and tansy. Flies hate mint, cloves, eucalyptus and shoo-fly plant. Weevils don't like bay. Pennyroyal is hard to beat for getting rid of insects. It is one of very few herbs that can actually kill them. Armed with this knowledge it's a simple matter to claim your home as your own and banish unwanted squatters.

minimize moths

Herb sachets (see page 95) are an excellent way of keeping moths out of your clothes. If you prefer, you can sprinkle the crushed, dried herbs into the bottom of drawers and then lay a piece of muslin or linen over the top. Every year you just vacuum out the old herbs and add fresh. Rosemary is the herb traditionally placed in chests of books and clothing to keep away moths but there are many herbs which moths don't like. The secret to repelling moths is to use herbs that you like the smell of on your clothes, rather than having to put up with the lingering smell of moth balls. There are many traditional recipes for moth-repelling herb sachets.

▲ shoo-fly
► pennyroyal

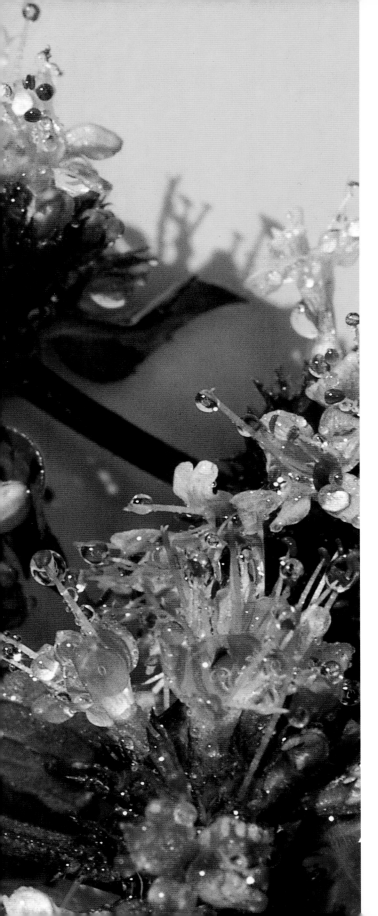

spicy protection

To keep insects out of the wardrobe and make your clothes smell delicious, try pomanders. Elizabethan women hung pomanders in elaborately jewelled cases around their neck or from their belt to ward off illness and unpleasant smells. Their pomanders were often made from balls of ambergris, a musky-smelling substance found washed up on the shore. We now know that it comes from the stomach of the sperm whale, but the substance was a complete mystery to ancient perfumiers. A ball of precious ambergris would be placed into the jewelled case on a bed of carefully chosen aromatic herbs.

The pomanders we make today are meant to suggest a little of the Elizabethan style but are far too big to hang around your neck! I tie mine with gold or silver ribbon and add a few beads or tassels to try to recapture some of the grandeur originally given to them and hang them in cupboards, wardrobes and small rooms.

orange and clove pomander

▶ *small thin-skinned orange*
▶ *cloves*
▶ *1 tsp powdered cinnamon*
▶ *1 tsp powdered orris root*
▶ *narrow ribbon*
▶ *more ribbon, beads, etc, to decorate*

Tie a narrow ribbon twice around an orange so that it is divided into four sections. Push the cloves into the skin of the orange (you may find it easier to make holes with a darning needle first) until you have neatly covered all four quadrants. Then roll the orange in the cinnamon and orris root, patting the powder in well. Wrap in greaseproof paper and leave in a cool dry place for five to six weeks, or two weeks in a warm, dry place like an airing cupboard. Dust off the powder, replace the ribbon with something more dazzling, and hang it in the wardrobe or in a linen cupboard.

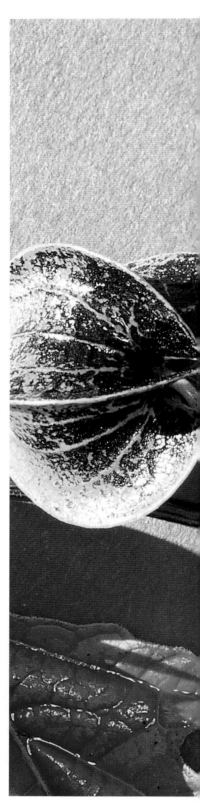

bug beaters

So having expelled all those insects from your house, what do you do when you go out in the garden or take a walk in the countryside? Herbs make good outdoor insect repellents for skin and clothes and the repellents are easy to make, too. But you need to reapply them often as the volatile oils, which make them effective, dissipate quickly. A note of caution. Essential oils can exert a powerful effect on the body. Don't use insect repellents containing them every day. Also, do not use pennyroyal if you are pregnant as it can increase the risk of miscarriage.

outdoor entertaining

Cooking and eating outdoors on a hot summer evening is enormously soothing – until insects gate-crash the party. Hang bunches of sage near where you are going to eat, particularly in trees you might like to sit beneath. Most insects don't like sage.

Herbs were traditionally tossed on to the open fire of the home to discourage insects. Doing this gives off wonderful aromas. Throw herbs into a barbecue or bonfire by tossing a handful of sage, rosemary, camomile, rue, lavender or pennyroyal on to the burning embers while you eat and you can 'fumigate' the whole area.

insect repellents for outdoors

Mosquitoes, midges and gnats	◆ Dilute a few drops of lavender or citronella essential oil in ½ cup of olive or almond oil and rub on the skin. ◆ Make a strong infusion of elderflowers (3-4 teaspoons of dried elderflowers to a cup of boiling water, steep for 10-15 minutes and strain) and use this as a wash on the skin.
Insects – in general	◆ In an emergency, grab a handful of fresh lemon balm, pennyroyal or basil and rub them straight on to the skin, *or* rub a peeled, halved onion over your skin. (Unfortunately this also repels the occasional person too.)
Insect-repellent spray	◆ Mix ½ cup of isopropyl alcohol with ½ cup water. Then add ½ teaspoon each of essential oils of pennyroyal, lavender and rose geranium. Put into a spray bottle, shake well and spray on to clothing. (Check that it doesn't stain your clothes first.)

► shoo-fly

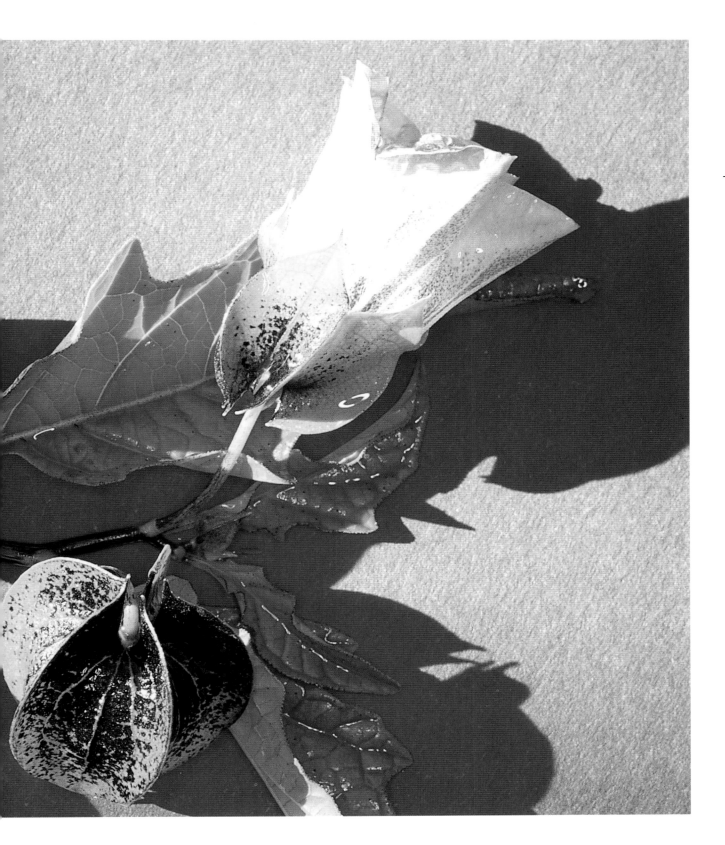

kitchen gardening

The simplest way of all to reap the health-enhancing rewards of plants is to eat them ...

Cook with herbs. Drop them raw into your salads. Garnish every dish with them. If you don't have room for a full-blown herb garden outside, then grow your herbs in containers indoors. These days, you can even buy them fresh in pots from the supermarket for use straight away.

inner garden

Growing herbs on your window ledges helps keep flies and other insects out of the kitchen (see page 103), as well as providing you with fresh herbs for cooking and making tea. Herbs famous for growing easily indoors include parsley, chives, dill, coriander and marjoram; but don't be afraid to try growing any herb indoors. The one plant I have always failed with is basil, which just happens to be my favourite culinary plant. I can never grow it in winter, nor indoors. But maybe you will be luckier. Every house (and every gardener) is unique and will suit different plants.

Sow your seeds directly into pots and take cuttings from your own and other people's gardens. By the way, thyme gathered from the side of a hill and kept in the house was traditionally used to conjure up fairies, so grow it indoors and you might get unexpected visitors.

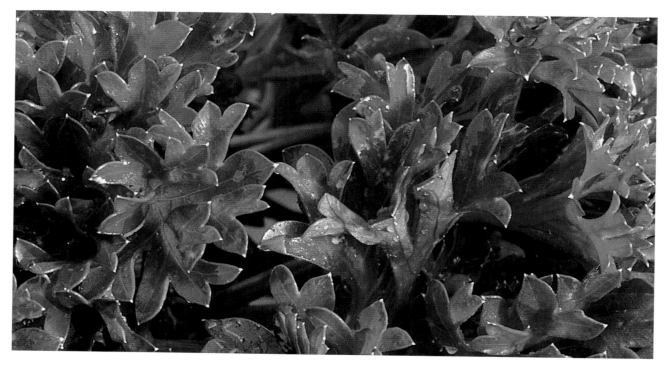

▲ parsley

One of the best things about growing herbs indoors is being able to smell them. I put them in places where I am likely to brush past them when opening windows or going through doorways, and where I can easily reach out and rub a leaf between my fingers. When you do this, plants love it and grow bigger and stronger – they really do!

creative herbs

When you think of all the wonderful uses herbs have been put to over the centuries it's a pity that the only thing some of us ever do with them is add them to cooking. Herbs have been used for decoration since the first time a human noticed they were pretty. They have been put around hats, woven into baskets, made into garlands to twist around the beams of village halls at weddings, tucked into button holes, threaded through hair: the list is endless. Use your imagination, you may be surprised at how many delightful things you can do with them.

For instance, cut a handful of rosemary or thyme stems and leaves, tie it into a short, tight bunch and use it as a basting brush. It won't melt like a plastic one, and it will release some of its volatile oils into whatever you are cooking. Or how about making a table decoration?

fresh table decoration

Get a brick of florist's foam (from your local florist), soak it in water, and stand it on an attractive plate. Take short stems of any fresh herbs you have to hand and push them into the foam until it is covered. My favourite herb for this is rosemary as its spiky leaves look really spectacular. I love it best when it is in flower. Legend has it that rosemary flowers were once white until one day the Virgin Mary threw her blue cloak over a bush to dry. The flowers were dyed with the colour of the cloth and have remained so to this day.

You can use just one herb or, if you prefer, blend textures and colours to make a spectacular centre piece. Investigate what shapes and sizes of foam your florist has – you can get cones, tubes, balls, and of course you can cut out your own shapes.

light fantastic

A lovely way to light a table for dinner is to use candles and lamps made from shells and scented with essential oils. Make shell candles that are deliciously perfumed. I make them from little shells I pick up on the beach and fill with candle wax and a wick. I melt the wax in a double-boiler and add a couple of drops of essential oil before pouring it into the shells so that they release the gentlest fragrance when lit. The shells can get hot so I place little groups of them around the table on small plates.

Alternatively, use oil in the shells to make tiny oil lamps. These are simply beautiful. Again I make them from shells found here and there. They get very hot so are best put on heat-proof plates or trays.

Stand the shells in a little blue-tac or Plasticine on your plate so that their open ends can act as a bowl. Put a wick inside the shells so that about 6 mm (¼ in) pokes out of the top (use candle wick or rub about a 5 cm (2 in) length of ordinary white household string with a wax candle). Fill the shell to just below its lip with any kitchen oil – olive or peanut, for instance – and a drop or two of essential oil. Light the wick, and you have the most delicate, romantic lamp imaginable.

after dinner mitts

After your meal, what could be better than relaxing with a cup of steaming peppermint tea. A friend of mine, Priscilla Palmer, has the most wonderful herb garden, called Willow Tree, in Christchurch, New Zealand. While visiting her recently she gave me a hot cup of tea in a glass which looked fabulously elegant but which, of course, was too hot for me to pick up and drink out of. Her solution was so simple I laughed out loud. Mug mitts. A mug mitt is a pretty oblong of fabric filled with herbs that wraps around a hot mug to protect your hands. In the process, the heat makes it release even more delicious fragrance.

You can make mitts from quilted fabric, or put your own wadding or further layers of fabric inside, then put a flat herb sachet inside this. Alternatively, use a thick fabric and fill your mitt with mung beans and dried herbs to make a little bean bag. The really fun bit is matching the right herb in the mitt with the tea in the mug!

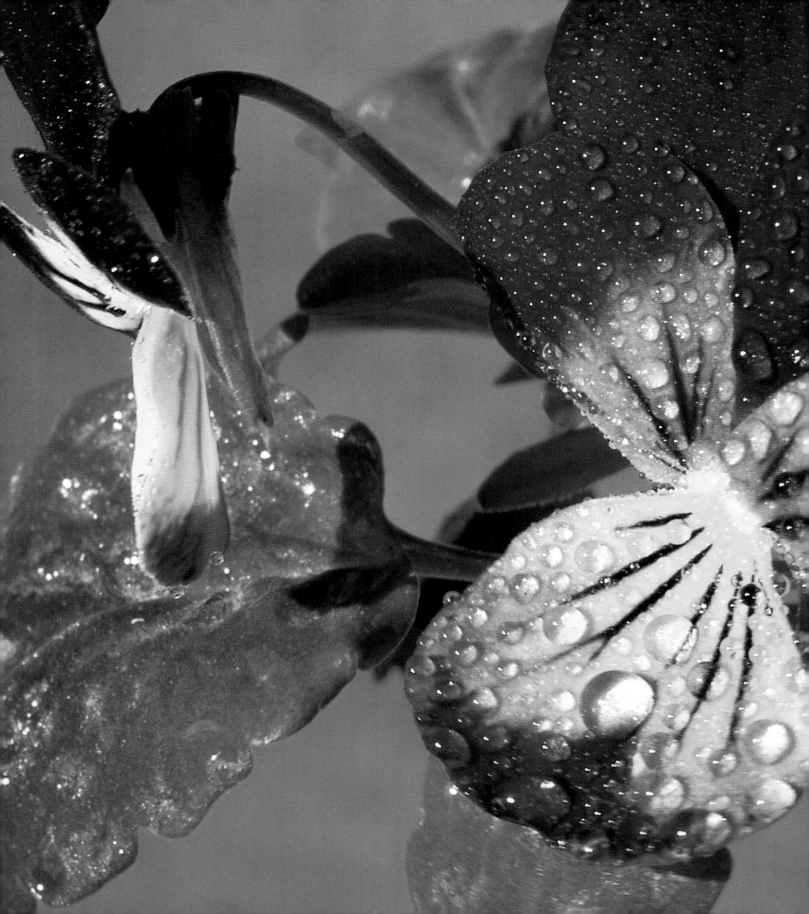

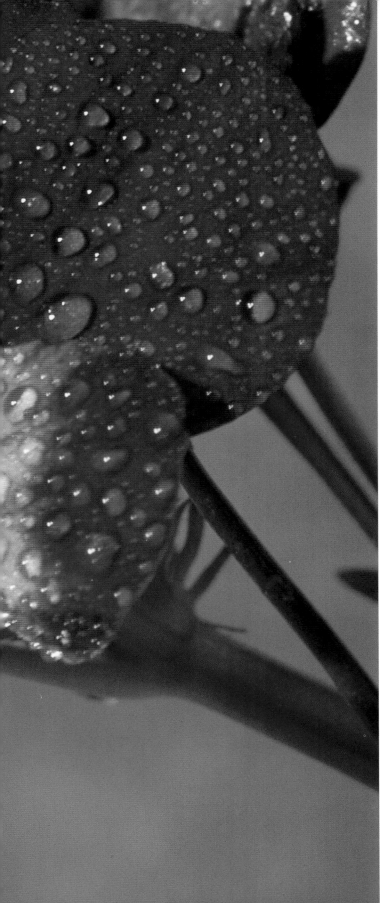

Soothing 5

Nowhere is the sacred power of plants more evident than in the help they offer us by countering the negative effects of stress. Herbs can help clear everything from anxiety to depression, addiction to sleeplessness - even burnout. The loving energy of plants pours forth in abundance whenever we need it most.

◄ heartsease

make stress a friend

Stress is by no means all bad. It brings a sense of challenge and adds spice to life ...

That is so long as your body is balanced and you are able to move at will from a dynamic and expansive stress state into a deeply relaxed restorative one. The trouble is that most of us get stuck in stress. We don't know how to get down when we need to. That is why we develop stress-related problems.

There are two approaches to good stress management using herbs. The first is a long-term strategy. You can call on specific plants such as ginseng, Siberian ginseng, astragalus and fo-ti to build up your adaptive energy – the kind of stamina that enables you to deal with stressors of all kinds long-term without suffering physical or psychological damage from them. These plants are known as adaptogenic because of their ability to strengthen the whole organism. They help protect against degeneration in the body. Many have also shown themselves in laboratory experiments to increase the life-span of animals.

The second approach to handling stress well is to call on plants that balance your brain and total metabolic chemistry and help you eliminate your specific symptoms. Herbal help works best when you do both. Not only can you clear troubling states and symptoms like depression, exhaustion, addiction, anxiety and sleeplessness, plant friends may even be able to help you turn your whole life around. With this dual method you can learn to make a friend of stress not just now but for the rest of your life. Remember, however, that herbs can sometimes take their time to kick in, so be patient and rest assured the help they offer lasts and lasts.

courage on call

Borage – the lovely *Borago officinalis* plant – was the first choice of Celtic warriors. They painted their bodies with it, drank borage wine and raced into battle naked. The belief that borage brings courage to those who eat and drink it is as old as recorded history. The Roman scholar Pliny called it euphrosinum and insisted that it lifted depression, while the Greek Dioscorides wrote in his *De Materia Medica* that borage 'cheers the heart and lifts depressed spirits'.

I use this herb in foods to help keep my spirits high. I toss a handful of leaves into the pot when I am making soup stock. I add its flowers and young leaves – which have a cucumber-like flavour – to my salads. You will find the gorgeous little borage flowers candied on the top of expensive cakes in Europe. I have never made borage wine but it is on my list of things to experiment with in the future. Borage does not dry well. Neither does it freeze, so use it fresh in your foods and make tea from its leaves and flowers. You can grow this lovely plant in pots indoors. Its tiny hairs and delicate flowers soften my heart. The borage flower alone is uplifting. It is almost too beautiful to touch.

▶borage

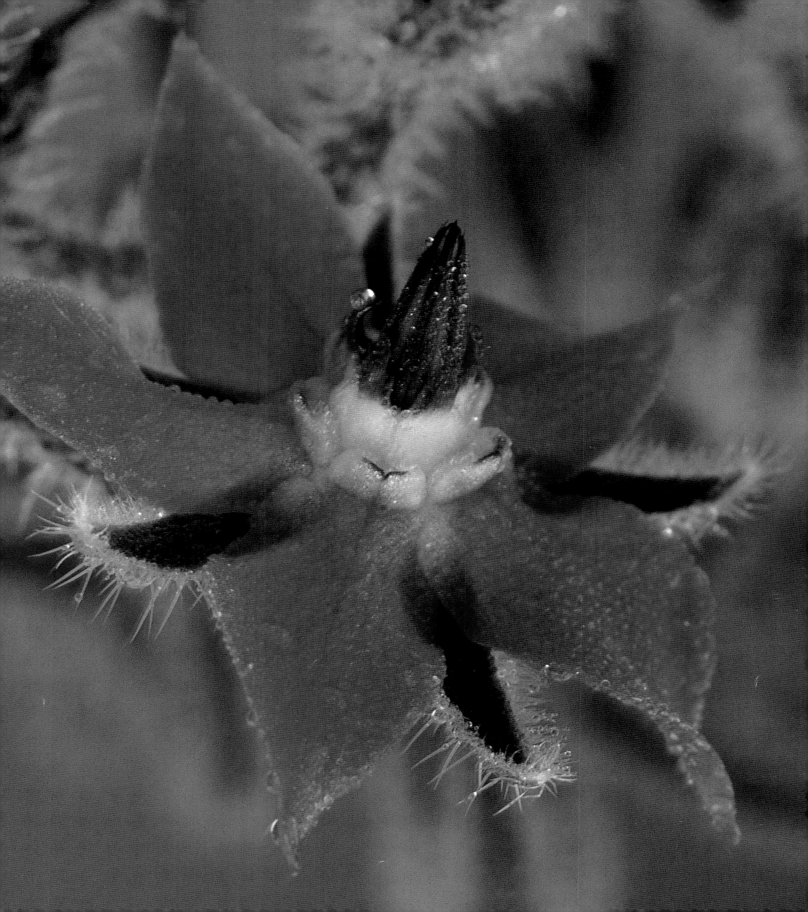

gathering power

A doctor, I.I. Brekhman – who as far back as the forties was studying the connection between stress and immune functions used the word to describe a very special group of plants such as Fo-ti, astragalus, the Ayurvedic plant combination tirphala, and Siberian ginseng. When taken over a long period of time these adaptogens have the ability to strengthen adaptation energy. Dr Hans Selye – who first defined stress in relation to human health – describes adaptation energy as the energy we have to sustain an effort or deal with pressure without causing damage to the mind or body. All adaptogens support and increase adaptation energy. They act as tonics to the system. But not all tonics are adaptogens.

These are pretty remarkable characteristics. But there is even something more remarkable about the adaptogenic herbs. They bring balance to our various organs and systems. For instance, if your blood pressure is too high and you take ginseng for several weeks, an adaptogen will lower it. Amazingly, taken by someone whose blood pressure is too low, the same plant will raise his or her blood pressure. Adaptogens are strengtheners, normalizers, power builders. That is why they play such an important role in any stress-related condition.

This ability to push and pull in whatever direction is needed is something that only exists in natural remedies. No drug has it. In any stress-related condition – whether it be depression, exhaustion, or anxiety – you almost always have a depletion of life energy – what the Chinese call qi. The adaptogens help you restore it. Without re-establishing your basic vitality, every other measure you take will only have a stop-gap effect.

The most useful group of adaptogenic plants is ginseng. Take them long-term. Together with a good natural diet rich in fresh vegetables and sea plants, regular gentle exercise and some form of meditation or deep relaxation practised each day, they will rejuvenate your body and regenerate your life.

oriental cure-all

The most famous of all the adaptogens – and the plant Brekhman did his first long-term studies with – is ginseng. In Asia this root has been used as a powerful tonic and rejuvenator for more than 3,000 years. For the last 150 we have known about it in the West – that is ever since a botanist named it *Panax ginseng*. *Panax* means 'cure all'. Use ginseng to enhance athletic performance, increase endurance, improve alertness, revive flagging memory and improve concentration. Traditional Chinese medicine insists that long-term use of ginseng also helps protect from cancer and other forms of degeneration as well as preventing

To be classified as an adaptogen a plant needs to do three things:

◆ Help normalize bodily functions even when you are unwell.

◆ Raise overall, non-specific, resistance to disease and degeneration – what is called cell-mediated immunity.

◆ Be safe – completely harmless – even when taken for long periods.

premature ageing. In recent years most of these claims have been substantiated by scientific research worldwide. Ginseng works to balance and strengthen both the cardiovascular and central nervous systems, while its effect on the thymus and spleen helps boost the immune system.

Ginseng contains every major type of potentially bioactive compound known to man, such as vitamins, minerals, amino acids and proteins. It is also rich in the key to ginseng – ginsenosides – which appear to be the key to ginseng's beneficial effect on the nervous system. One of this plant's traditional uses has been in the control of diabetes. It helps maintain blood sugar levels and therefore stabilizes energy.

which one?

There are three different varieties of ginseng.

Panax ginseng is the most prized and most expensive. It is grown either in China (the best) or Korea and is known as ren shen. It is always best to go for this one if you can possibly afford it. Buy it as dried and powdered root in capsules, as an extract, a tincture, or as the root itself, either whole or sliced, which you can then chew. Ginseng's potency depends a lot on where it is grown, how it is cultivated, stored and prepared. Be sure you have a good quality supply. My favourite way of taking ginseng is as a tea. You will need to take it for several weeks to gain the full benefit of its strengthening, balancing and restorative powers.

Panax quinquefolius is known as American ginseng or xi yang shen. It is mostly used for fevers and to treat exhaustion from chronic wasting diseases. It also helps to strengthen the lungs.

Panax notoginseng is really a pseudo-ginseng known as san qi in China. There they use it to stop pain and bleeding. It was used a lot by the Viet Cong during the Vietnam war to speed recovery from wounds.

The plant *Eleutherococcus senticosus* bears the common name 'Siberian ginseng', yet it is not a ginseng at all. Like fo-ti, it is another of the Chinese qi tonic herbs used by athletes in the West to enhance prowess and stamina. It has ginseng-like adaptogenic effects however. It builds strength, enhances immunity and helps restore normal blood pressure and helps protect the liver from stress and the damage caused by toxic build-up. I take between ½ and 1 gram of Siberian ginseng in capsule form three times a day over several weeks for the best results. You can also take *Eleuthrococcus* as a tincture: take ½ to 1 teaspoon, three times a day.

ginseng tea

▶ *1 tsp dried ginseng root*
▶ *1 cup water*

Put the dried root into a pan with the water. Bring it to the boil and simmer for 10 minutes. Strain and drink. Alternatively, use a good brand of granulated ginseng which has been carefully processed to preserve its power yet made to dissolve in hot water (see Resources). I put two packets to each cup and drink it three or four times a day during periods of heavy stress or when I have allowed myself to become chronically tired.

Caution:

Ginseng can sometimes cause insomnia, and if you have cardiovascular disease, it is best used under the direction of a good health-care practitioner. Do not take it if you are pregnant, and don't give it to children as some of the ginsenosides are chemically similar to some steroidal hormones that might possibly have an effect on a child's growth or development.

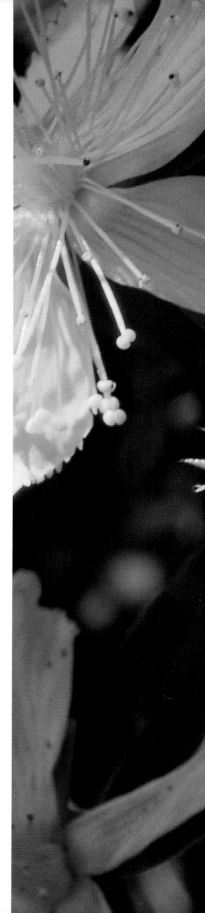

beating the blues

Depression can be a killer.
I know. I suffered from it badly in my
early twenties ...

I was born with a tendency towards depression and I am familiar with the deep sadness, feelings of shame and helplessness, the terrible fatigue coupled with not being able to sleep to relieve it, the poor concentration and strange shifts in appetite. I have learned a lot about handling it over the years. There are many causes of depression – some are of the body and some of the psyche. I don't think you can separate the two. Just as body and mind feed each other in producing the dark, seemingly endless blues which can set in at any period of your life, the herbs you call on for help will improve both body and spirit. When you feel depressed you can feel anxious as well. Many of the plants that are effective in lifting the blues help to clear fear and anxiety too.

deep cleansing

Where you find depression, you almost always find a mass of creative energy, which – for one reason or another – has remained blocked. This can make you feel impotent and helpless. You also often find a tendency to live life by other people's rules rather than your own – that is from the depths of your own soul. Indeed, when depression is deep and debilitating enough, you can even come to feel you have no soul to live from. Deep cleansing your body is an important step in releasing blocked creative energy and restoring the biochemical balance that helps wash the blues away.

Use the Herbal Cleanse on pages 40-51, but take it further. When the cleanse is finished, try following a long-term way of eating based on fresh vegetables – many of them raw – and good quality proteins from fish, organic meat, free-range chicken, eggs and tofu. Avoid milk products including milk itself, yoghurt and cheese (butter is OK because it is a fat and it is the milk protein that tends to cause problems for people prone to depression). Also cut out wheat and anything made from wheat flour such as pasta, breakfast cereals, breads and biscuits and, finally, make highly processed convenience foods a thing of the past. It was just such a diet – one in which at least 50-75% of the foods I ate were raw – that cleared my own deep depression in my twenties.

Meanwhile, turn your attention to herbs and find out just how much they can do to rebalance brain chemistry, strengthen your body and clear your mind. Use an adaptogen to raise your body's energy, strengthen immunity and balance metabolic functions (see pages 114-15). Then call on the healing powers of some of the best natural antidepressants: St John's wort, rosemary, California poppy and ginkgo.

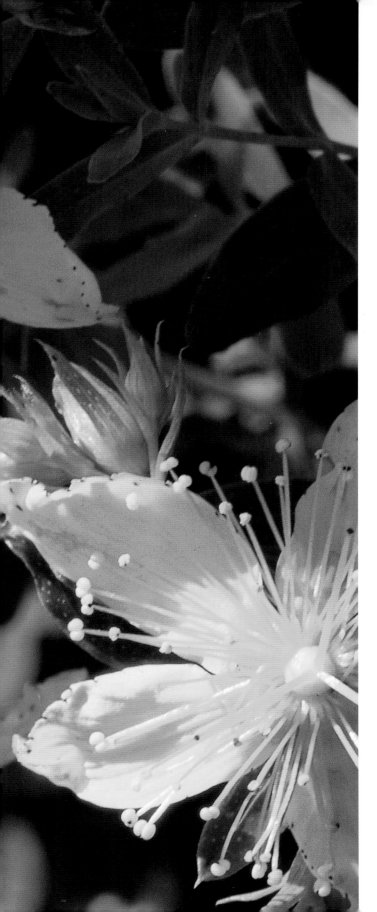

bright as sunlight

Bright as morning sun, the yellow flowers and dancing leaves of St John's wort (*Hypericum perforatum*) bring balance and joy. This plant may be slow to act, but its effects are deep and long-lasting. St John's wort is nature's answer to Prozac. Every part of this joyous herb yields uplifting power – its leaves, its shoots, its glorious yellow flowers. Even the way it grows seems to celebrate life. Use St John's wort to banish anxiety, bring light into the dark depths of depression, and to transform difficult times – loss of a job, of a lover, or of sense of purpose – into times of power.

Recently, St John's wort has attracted a lot of attention. Twenty-three random clinical trials have shown this plant is just as effective, if not more so, as standard antidepressant drugs. Yet it comes without negative side-effects. Like antidepressant drugs, St John's wort increases the levels of serotonin, the 'feel-good' neurotransmitter, in your brain. In Germany alone, 600,000 prescriptions are written for this plant each year.

Externally, St John's wort is a valuable anti-inflammatory remedy. It boasts antiviral and antibacterial activity and speeds the healing of wounds and burns. What is already known of this herb is astonishing enough, but the best may be yet to come. Excitingly, it is proving itself to be a promising treatment for Chronic Fatigue Syndrome. Its greatest promise may be as a treatment of AIDS.

The bright yellow flowers of St John's wort contain a red oil called hypericin, which is antiviral and probably mood enhancing. Many studies show that it is whole

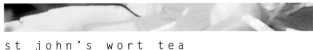

st john's wort tea

◎ 1-2 tsp dried St John's wort
◎ 1 cup boiling water

Steep the herb in the water for 10-15 minutes, strain, and drink three times a day.

◉ st john's wort

plant extracts, however, rather than hypericin alone that have the best antidepressant effects. One of the most effective ways to use St John's wort for depression is as a tincture. Take 1 teaspoon of St John's wort tincture in a little water three times a day. When used as an antidepressant it should be taken for at least a month before seeing results. A lucky few people, however, respond right away.

Pick the flowers, leaves and stems of St John's wort while the plant is in flower. Dry them quickly as you want to preserve the red oil in the flowers. You can also make the dried flowers into a useful oil for first aid (see page 34).

california bright lights

California poppy is the best anxiety-calming herb I know and it works quickly and in only a few hours. Its watery sap has long been used by Native Americans to relieve toothache. It relieves pain, relaxes spasms and warms your body, but don't worry, it is not a narcotic, only a gentle sedative and tranquillizer so safe that herbalists give it to children. Neither does it depress the central nervous system. The usual dose of tincture is 1 teaspoon to half a glass of water taken twice a day in the afternoon and evening. I like to combine tincture of golden California poppy (*Eschscholzia californica*) with that of St John's wort – in equal parts – to lift the blues.

invigorate with rosemary

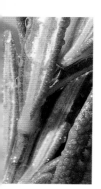

Rosmarinus officinalis grows just about everywhere. Who would ever suspect that it is one of the most useful herbs you will ever find for lifting the blues. The strong and sturdy plant is an excellent tonic and all-round stimulant. It raises spirits and energizes the body, clearing apathy, nervous exhaustion and digestive disturbances associated with anxiety. Rosemary has a longstanding reputation for strengthening the memory too. That is why Greek scholars wore garlands of rosemary when they took exams. Rosemary is also rejuvenating and strengthens capillaries and collagen in the skin.

In the fourteenth century, 72-year-old Izabella Queen of Hungary was crippled with rheumatism. She used masses of Hungary Water

Cautions:

In a few people St John's wort causes mild nausea, stomachache, depressed appetite, tiredness, and in even fewer still, sensitivity to sunlight. It shouldn't be taken during pregnancy. If you are already taking antidepressant drugs do not stop taking your medication without consulting your doctor.

Never take California poppy while taking MAO inhibitor drugs without your doctor's permission.

► california poppy

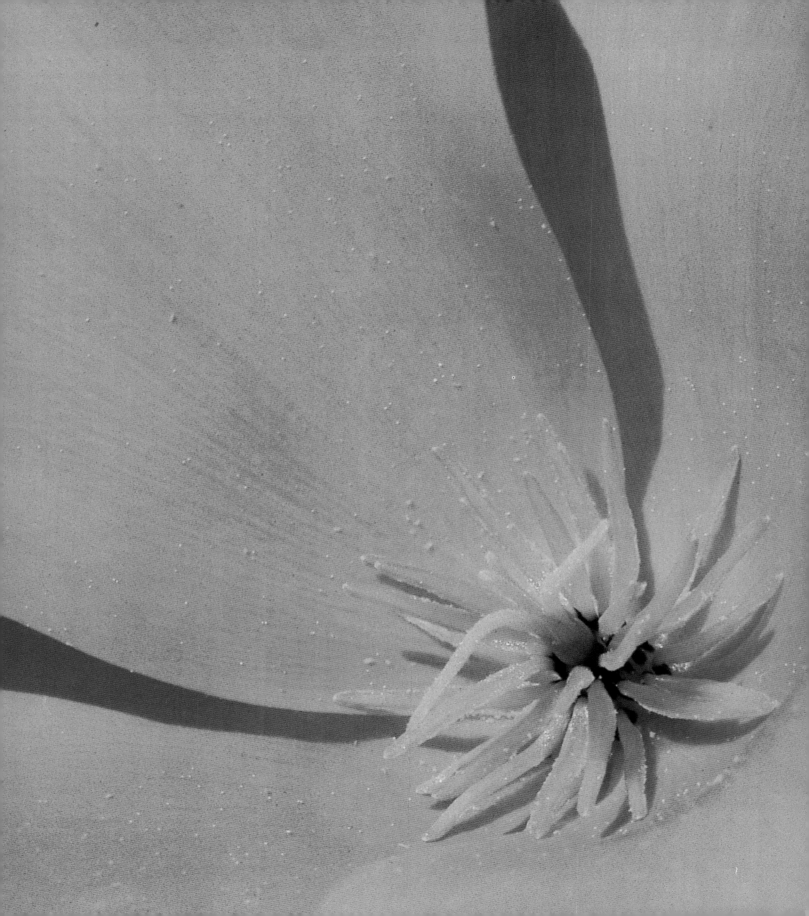

(rosemary leaves macerated in alcohol) and regained her youth so well that the king of Poland proposed to her.

One of the first to be distilled, essential oil of rosemary can help clear a fuzzy head with ease. You can use the fresh leaves or the essential oil in steam inhalations for exhaustion and shattered nerves. Meanwhile, rosemary tea is bracing and wonderfully uplifting.

ginkgo clears the cobwebs

The beautiful leaves from *Ginkgo biloba* – also known as the maidenhair tree – improve circulation all over the body, including the brain. Its seeds were sent to Europe in the 1720s from Japan and China. The Chinese use the ginkgo seeds but research in the West tends to concentrate on the leaves. They contain ginkgolides, unknown in any other plant. These phyto-chemicals block blood platelet activating factors. In doing so they inhibit all sorts of allergic responses.

Meanwhile, ginkgo's flavonoids do wonders to improve circulation to the brain. Recent studies show that this long-standing oriental herbal remedy can help clear depression too. Gingko increases the rate at which information is transmitted at the level of nerve cells. This helps depression in many people, thanks to its enhancing the flow of neurotransmitters in the brain. An effective anti-depressant dose in one study where gingko was used to counter depression was 240 milligrams of the powdered herb in capsule form a day. It can take six to eight weeks to experience the full effects of ginkgo.

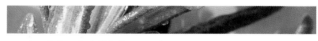

spirit lifting tea

▶*1 tbsp fresh rosemary leaves or 1-2 tsp dried*
▶*boiling water*

Put the rosemary leaves into a warmed pot and pour boiling water over them. Replace the lid to prevent the aromatic vapours from being wasted. Leave to brew for 5 minutes. Drink hot.

▶ ginkgo

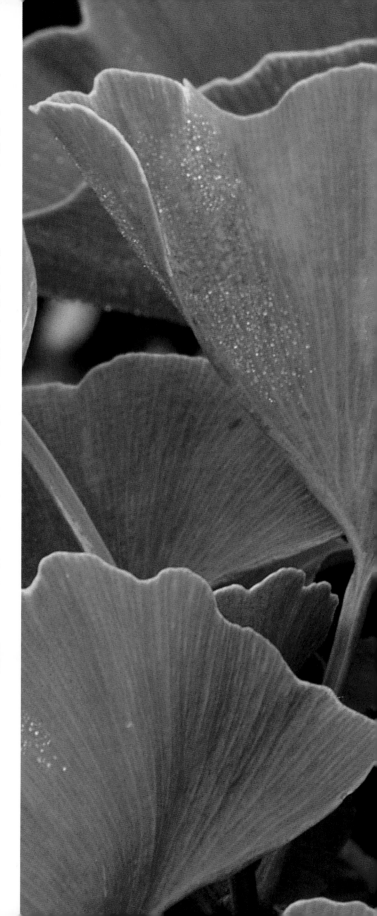

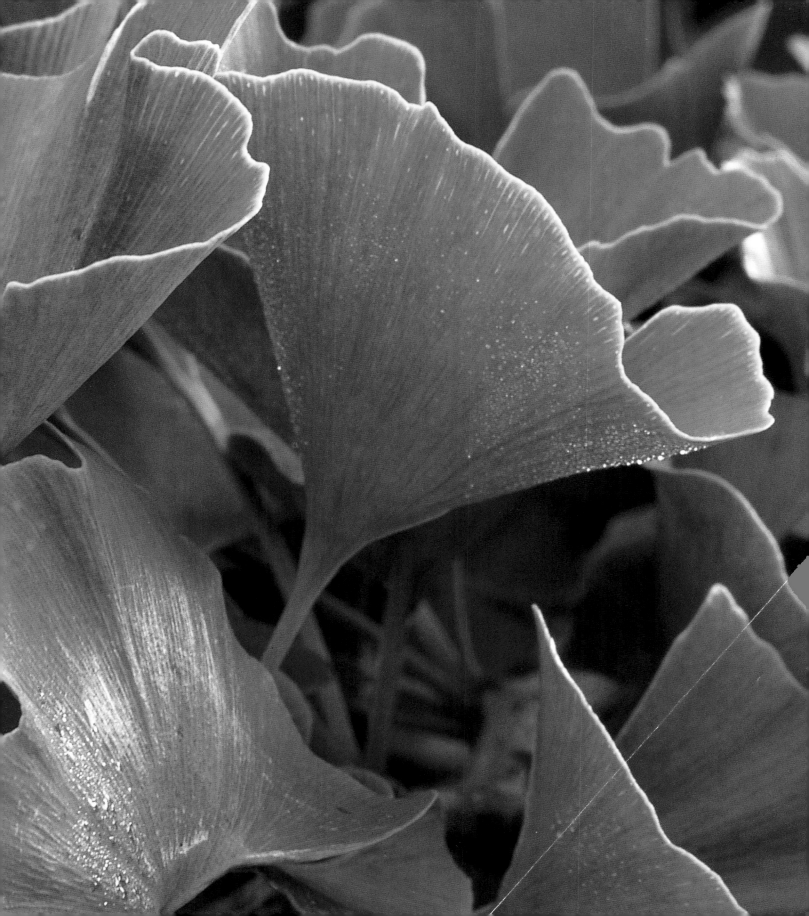

help for anxiety

Chronic anxiety is another mental
state I am far more familiar with than
I would like to be ...

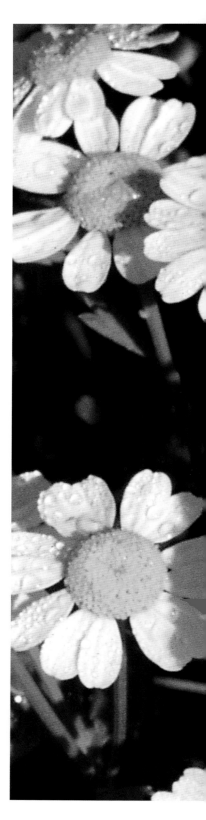

To me it seems unfair that depression, which brings you down, is often accompanied by anxiety that makes you feel helpless and unsafe in the world. When anxiety raises its ugly head in my life I begin to suspect that something deep within me is trying to be born. Some neglected or ignored part of me is attempting to break though the routine existence which, because I feel familiar and reasonably safe with it, I tend to cling to. Knowing that most likely this is happening for my own good, to help me grow, doesn't make it any easier to deal with. It is in such circumstances that I turn to plants for help: camomile, kava kava, motherwort, valerian, borage (for courage), hops, lemon balm or skullcap. Here are some of the ways I use them.

camomile

I love the way these tiny flowers calm the central nervous system and there are many ways to use them. Gather German camomile (*Matricaria chamomilla*) or Roman camomile (*Anthemis nobilis*) flowers during the summer months making sure that all the dew has evaporated. Then lay them on paper to dry and store them in a dark cupboard. You can then use the dried herbs for all manner of things, such as in a muslin bag in a bath (see page 128). Alternatively, put essential oil of camomile into a diffuser while working and a few drops in your bath with the dried flowers.

lemon balm

Calming and sedative, this lovely plant (*Melissa officinalis*) is so mild even children can use it. In addition to its anti-anxiety properties, it helps lift depression and also calms digestive upsets. Use the essential oil of lemon balm – five drops of it neat – in the bath. Or make an infusion of a tablespoon of the fresh leaves (you can substitute dried leaves if you like but it doesn't taste anywhere near as good) and drink it hot or cold with a slice of fresh lemon or lime. Make massage oil of it too: dilute 5 to 10 drops of the pure essential oil in a tablespoon of almond or grapeseed oil. Rub it on your body when you feel tense or troubled.

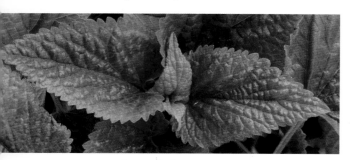

▲ lemon balm   ► camomile

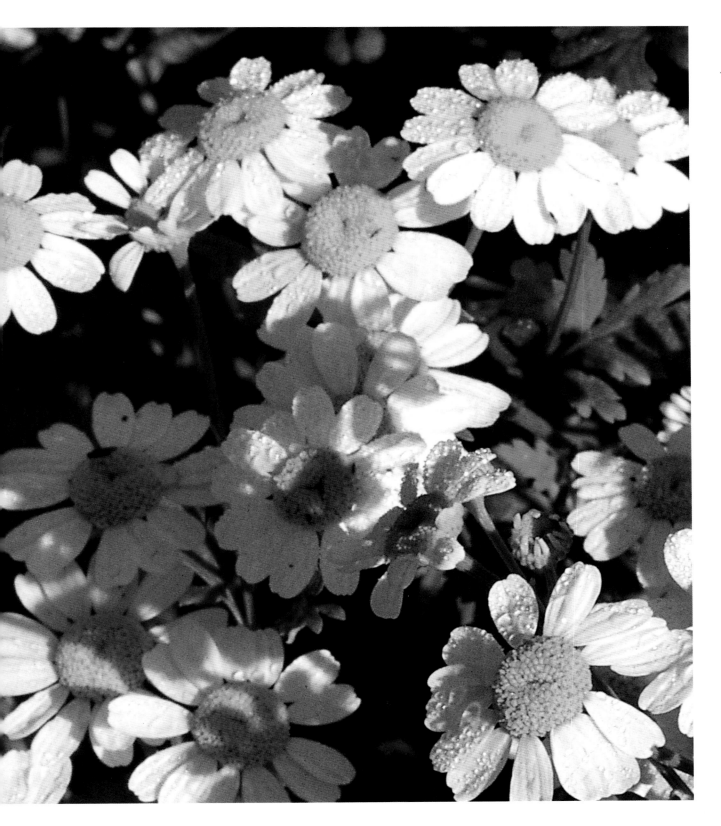

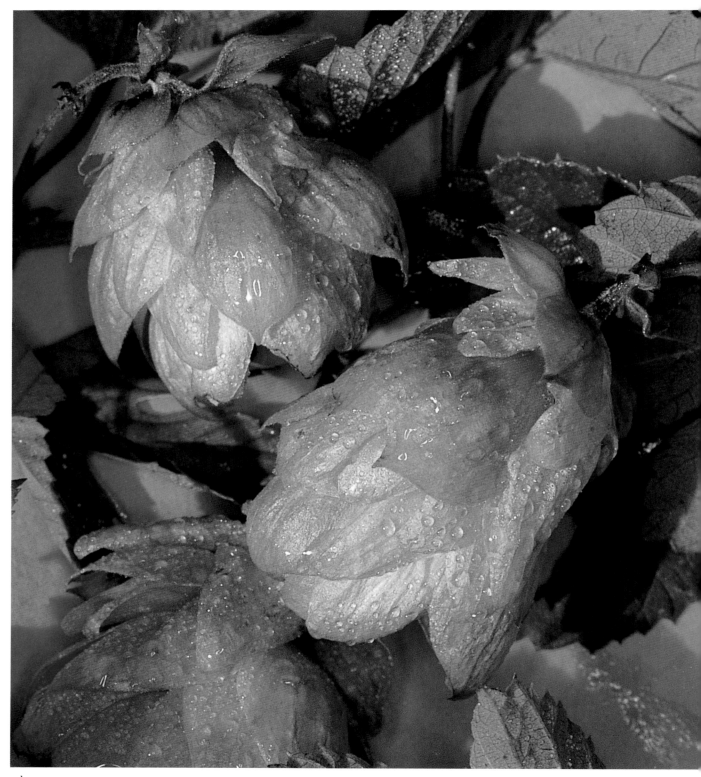

▲ hops

healing hops

The flowers of a female hop plant (*Humulus lupulus*) are called strobiles. They are the plant part used for healing. And they have both a sedative and a tonic effect thanks to volatile oils, valerianic acid, flavonoids, phyto-hormones and tannins. Hops even work as aphrodisiacs. They are ideal for restoring balance to frayed nerves.

hop tea

▶ *2-3 tsp fresh or dried hop flowers*
▶ *1 cup boiling water*

To allay anxiety, make an infusion of hop strobiles by steeping the flowers in the water for 5 minutes. You can use freeze- or air-dried hops in place of fresh flowers.

the root of mind bending

Kava kava (*Piper methysticum*) is another of my favourite chill-out herbs. It is a consciousness-altering root with immediate effect. In Tonga, this root forms the locus of the warm and wonderful kava ceremony, which unites people in good will and relaxation the way no other plant I have ever known can. Natives gather the kava roots, dry them and pound them. Then they place them in a beautiful wooden kava bowl, mix them with water and spit into the mixture. This has the effect of making the alkaloids in the plant more psychoactive.

Kava kava is the quickest-acting natural anti-depressant and relaxant known to man. Just as it traditionally unifies the tribe, kava kava unifies the person – banishing the sense of fragmentation that is common to modern life. Kava kava can also be a great quick fix for the soul. It brings a sociable relaxation and contentment allowing conversation to flow – just like alcohol, but without the aggression or loss of responsibility. Kava sharpens rather than dulls the senses and leaves you with no hangover.

Calming to both mind and body, kava promotes sleep. And the body does not seem to become 'tolerant' to its effects so kava does not lose its power to help over time. There have been many trials to establish kava's ability to relieve anxiety. The most recent studies indicate that (taken in small doses) it can reduce anxiety significantly after one, two and four weeks of treatment without side-effects. A safe alternative to dangerous tranquillizers, sleeping pills and antidepressants, kava is used by some of the largest pharmaceutical companies as a basis for medicines designed to treat anything from urinary tract infections to arthritis as well as nervous disorders of all kinds. Menopausal symptoms are sometimes relieved by taking regular doses of kava – and not just those associated with stress and anxiety either. Kava improves mood and cools hot flushes.

It is the kava root that holds the plant's medicinal power. It appears that kava's relaxing properties derive from its oxygen-containing, lipid-like compounds that are known as lactones or pyrones. Six major kavalactones and a dozen minor ones have so far been identified. They may influence GABA, the neurotransmitter that calms the central nervous system. Some studies show that the kavalactones seem to act on the limbic system too, an ancient part of the brain which is considered to be the seat of instinct and emotion. It is the whole root of kava which has the greatest effect, not its isolated compounds. You can buy kava dried in capsules, as a tincture and as an extract. it is the extract form that I like the best.

kava bliss

◆ Take 1 teaspoon of extract of kava in a little water when you need to relax. You will feel it in your stomach within 2 minutes, in your brain with 5 minutes.

Caution:
High doses of potent kava products can reduce motor control and may even cause liver problems. It's not a good idea to drive or operate machinery if you have taken a high dose, so go easy. Persistent heavy use may also cause diarrhoea, lethargy and apathy in some people, or even a scaly skin condition. These conditions can be reversed by ceasing to take kava. Do not use kava kava and alcohol at the same time.

a passion for peace

The elaborate purple and white passionflower (*Passiflora incarnata*) takes its name from the passion of Jesus. According to medieval monks, in its centre you will find an echo of the cross on which the saviour died for the sins of the world. Roughly one-third of the population experiences regular insomnia. In the United States alone 10 million prescriptions for heavy duty sleeping pills are written each year. Passionflower can take many people through the transition from wakefulness into restful sleep without the sleeping-pill hangover in the morning. It has a sedative and mildly narcotic effect on the body.

The leaves carry the strength for deep relaxation and their action is immediate. You can use passionflower for nerve pain and hysteria. Passionflower is good for women who wrestle with nervous tension and for when nerves are edgy before periods or around the time of menopause. Passiflora's most active constituent 'passiflorine' appears to be similar in its chemical structure to morphine. It has analgesic and anti-spasmodic properties. It is helpful to asthma sufferers – especially when attacks are triggered by stress and tension. Collect passionflower leaves just before the flowers bloom and dry them gently. You can then make an infusion of them. You can also take passionflower as an extract or tincture.

passionflower infusion

▶ *1 tsp dried passionflower leaves*
▶ *1 cup boiling water*

Put the dried leaves in a tea pot and pour the water over them and steep for 15 minutes. Drink twice a day to ease anxiety, then take a third cup before bed to help you to sleep. Or you can use ½-1 teaspoon of tincture in a little water three times a day.

Caution:
It is probably best not to use passionflower when you need to be fully alert.

▶ passionflower

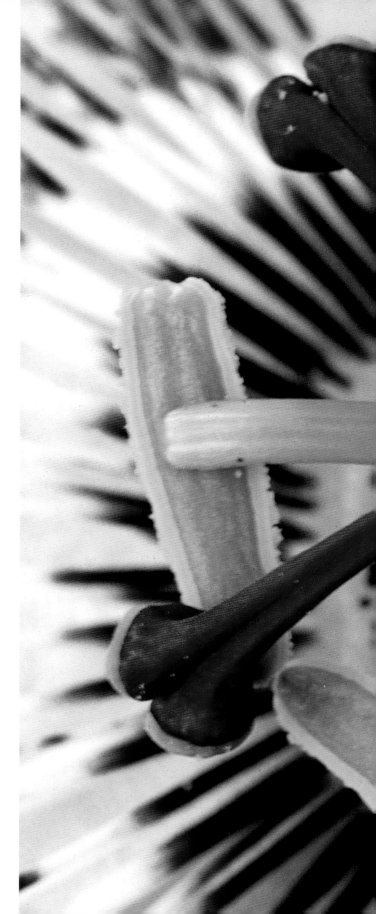

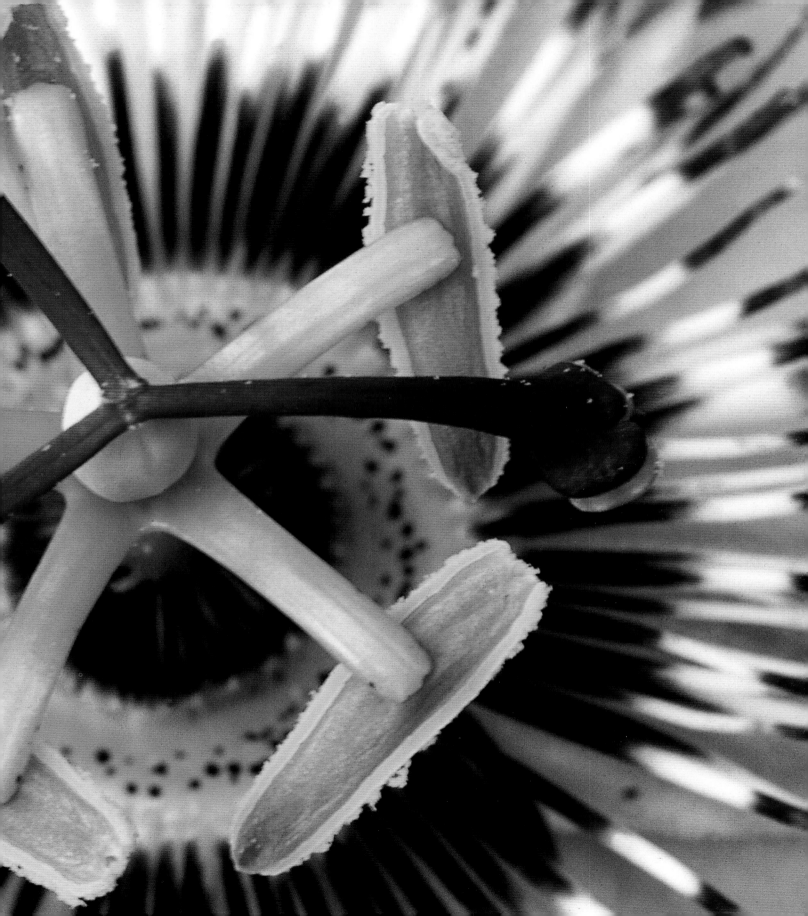

midnight soak

No matter how exhausted you may feel at the end of the day don't be tempted to just flop into bed unless you are relaxed ...

Sleep is something to be savoured and enjoyed, not something to dash yourself against. Taking a bath if you awaken in the night can be one of the most relaxing things you can do. The telephone is unlikely to ring, nor will anyone want you to do something for them. A herb bath to relax you deeply can be more of a treat than a remedy. Adding essential oils will also help: try 2-3 drops of lavender oil, camomile or neroli. Or put a drop of each on your pillow.

Water, fortified with plant essences, can soothe, heal, and relax a tense and weary body as well as lift a sagging spirit. When you step into the bath it is time to let go of all your cares. Bathing can be blissful but it is a serious business. The relaxation it brings restores energy and helps make whole a fragmented mind. Whenever you can, make bath-time a real performance in a warm bathroom filled with wonderful fragrance, soft music and gentle light. And before you even touch a tap, make sure that you have everything you need to hand: a loofah or hemp glove, towel, another towel to act as a head-rest, sea salt for rubs, Epsom salts, and herbs or oils of your choice.

it's in the bag

To prevent herbs sticking to the bath and to you; as well as clogging the plug-hole, create a sort of 'tea bag' by sewing up three sides of a 15 cm (6 in) square muslin bag. Put your herbs into it and sew up the last side. These bags can be used again and again so sewing a few is worth the investment in time. If you only want to use your herbs once, you can put them in the middle of a square of muslin, make a bundle of it and secure it with an elastic band. When you've done with it you can throw the herbs away and wash the muslin to be used again.

Toss a herb bag into your bath as you are running it, or make your bag with string or ribbon ties so it hangs under the flow from the hot tap. Leave it in the water for the first 5 minutes of your bath, then squeeze it out thoroughly and put it on the side. You can use the wet bag like a flannel to wash with. If this seems like too much effort you can even make a super-strong infusion of your herbs in a tea pot and pour this into the bath – it will have the same effect.

what a smoothie

A herb bath is an opportunity to pamper your skin with natural ingredients in the most luxurious way. Before you dip a foot in the water, however, try a sea salt scrub. If you think exfoliation means expensive preparatory body creams then think again. A handful of sea salt mixed with a little water rubbed all over your body will remove dead skin cells, soften your skin, and leave you glowing all over. There is nothing quite like the tingle of warm water on just-scrubbed skin! A salt rub taken before a herbal bath also increases the benefits of the herbs because it makes your skin more absorbent. A particularly delicious way to use a salt scrub is to mix a cup or two of your dried herbs – rosemary, peppermint, orange peel or camomile – into the salt. Fill a glass jar with your mixture and keep it in the bathroom, it looks and smells delicious.

bathroom essentials

The potency of essential oils is such that they work better highly diluted. They are perfect in the bath. Essential oils soothe a tired body and a troubled mind. As you breathe in their mood-enhancing qualities on the steam

blissful bags

To relax you
◆ Use 1½ cups of any of these dried herbs on their own, or a mixture of ½ cup each of two or three: camomile, comfrey, hyssop, juniper berries, lavender, lemon balm, mullein, passionflower, peppermint, slippery elm, valerian

To invigorate you
◆ Try any of these plants, or mix together ½ cup each of two or three: calendula, fennel, horseradish root, lavender, marjoram, mint, nettle, pine needles, rosemary, sage, thyme

To ease aching muscles
◆ Use a mixture of ½ cup each of two or three: crushed juniper berries, oregano, sage, strawberry leaves

To bathe tired feet
◆ Try a mixture of ½ cup each of two or three herbs in a comfortably hot foot bath: agrimony, burdock, ginger, lavender, bruised mustard seed, sage, witch hazel

perfect essences

To diffuse anger
◆ Ylang ylang, rose, camomile

To unlock resentment
◆ Rose

To cheer you up
◆ Hyssop, marjoram, sandalwood

To invigorate your mind
◆ Basil, peppermint, cypress, patchouli

To ease worry
◆ Lavender

To stop world-weariness
◆ Neroli, melissa, camphor

To make you feel stronger
◆ Camomile, jasmine, melissa

To soothe irritability
◆ Frankincense, marjoram, camomile, lavender

To relieve exhaustion
◆ Jasmine, rosemary, juniper, patchouli

To unknot anxiety
◆ Sage, juniper, basil, jasmine

you will absorb their healing properties through your skin. I have a collection of them which I keep in the bathroom and use often.

There are two ways of adding essential oils to a bath. You can put 2-3 drops of the pure essence into running water; or you can make a simple bath oil by adding 5 drops of essential oil to ¼ cup of carrier oil such as apricot or almond oil. Pour this mixture into the water 5 minutes after you have got into the bath. This gives your skin time to absorb some moisture. Otherwise the oil can cling to your skin as you get into the bath and act as a barrier. Your own home-made herb oils are also wonderful in the bath.

minimalist baths

A herb bath doesn't necessarily mean filling the bath with water and fully immersing yourself either. You might like to try a sitz bath. This can be great for healing lower back troubles and period pain. Simply put 15 cm (6 in) of warm water into the tub. Add your herbs (don't use essential oils, they might burn your skin in so little water) and sit in it for 10-15 minutes, keeping the top half of your body well wrapped up. Step out of the bath and wrap yourself in a towel – don't dry yourself with it. Go and lie down in a warm room for 20 minutes and soak up the chance to relax.

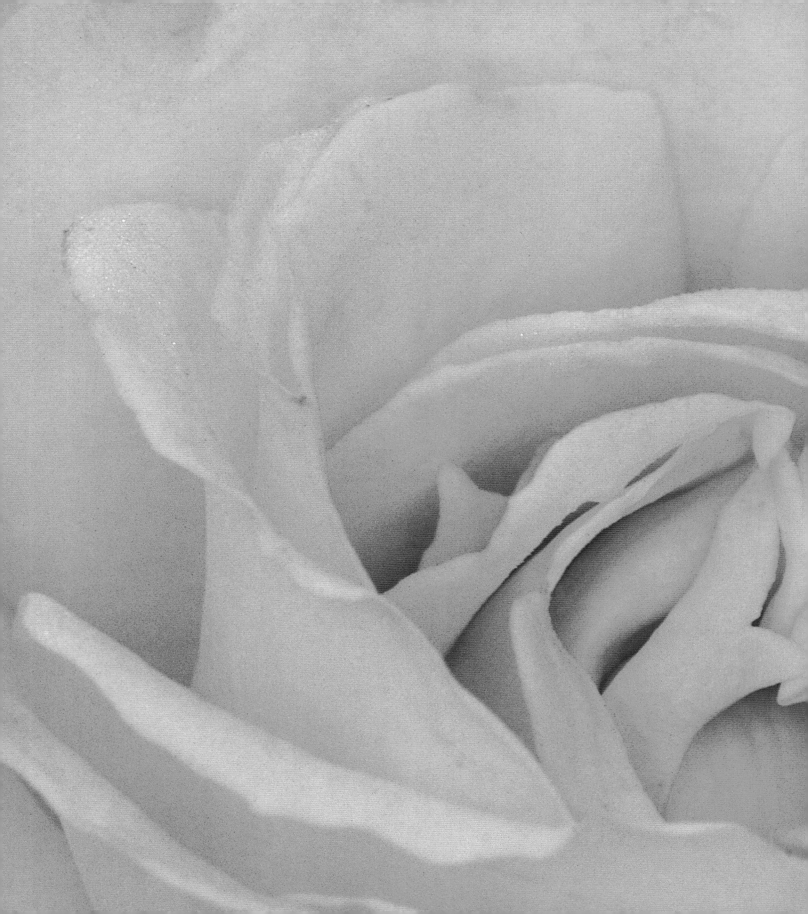

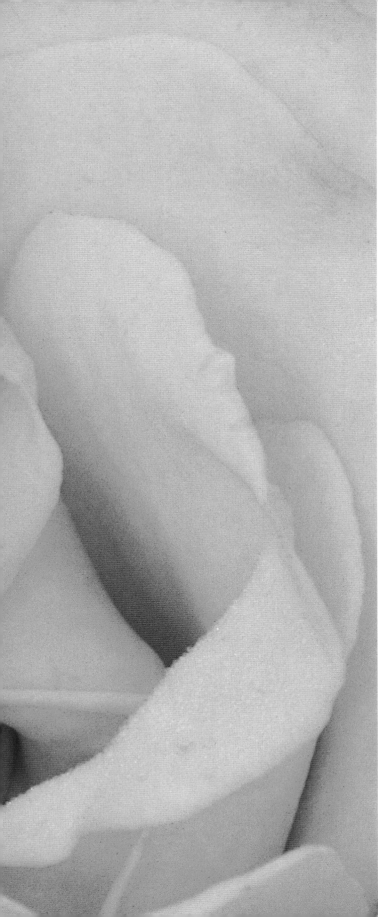

enhancing 6

Herbs revel in sacred beauty. It is fundamental to their nature. They love to be gathered tenderly and made a part of our day-to-day lives. Like the earth in which they grow, plants offer up their magnificence to deepen and expand the beauty in our own lives. They can make your body or your bath, your room or your morning more wonderful. Yet often the glory of a plant reaches far deeper - penetrating even the human soul with its splendour. Open yourself to such beauty. Your life will be filled with grace.

◄ rose

more than skin deep

It lives, it breathes ...

Your skin is far more than a superficial covering for your body. It is your largest organ. And, like your hair and nails, skin needs a good supply of vitamins, minerals, protein, essential fatty acids, trace elements and unrefined carbohydrates to keep it healthy and beautiful, sleek and smooth. Vitamin A, for instance, helps regulate the size and function of sebaceous glands in the skin and scalp, Vitamin E and the B-complex vitamins aid circulation in the skin and the transport of oxygen to the cells. Vitamins A, C, and E are vital antioxidants too. They help protect skin from premature ageing, sagging and wrinkling.

The minerals zinc, magnesium, iron, potassium and selenium can all be leached from your body if you eat a diet high in protein. They are just as important as the vitamins. Selenium preserves tissue elasticity. Zinc speeds up the process of skin healing and helps clear up blemishes. You need enough protein, of course, to keep your skin and hair glowing with health. In order to make proper use of your proteins you need to have sufficient enzymes to break them down into the amino acids your body uses for the formation of protein-based structures – such as hair. You also need enzymes to then build these amino acids into new skin and hair proteins. The function of many of these enzymes in your body depends on there being enough zinc available to act as a co-factor for them, and enough silicon to make them strong.

minerals matter

High-tech farming methods have destroyed so much of the organic matter in our soils that fruits and vegetables no longer contain a good quantity of minerals and trace elements. Commercial food processing wipes out much of what's left. Buy organically grown fruits and vegetables from well-established sources whenever you can. Herbs can help redress the balance. Take dandelion, for instance. Dandelion is rich in iron, silicon, magnesium, sodium, potassium, zinc, manganese, copper and phosphorus in an unbeatable synergistic balance. Put dandelion leaves in your salads (see page 71). Drink dandelion tea often (see page 44). It will help restore your body's lost minerals, and you will also be getting an extra dose of vitamins A, B, C and D into the bargain.

Silicon is another essential trace element. Our daily requirement is small, but unless we eat organically grown food and unless the soils they were grown on are rich in this element we simply don't get enough – often not even then. Silicon helps to bind minerals needed for strong nails, hair and bones. It is also essential to the production of the skin's connective tissues – collagen and elastin. The delicate horsetail plant is one of the world's earliest forms of plant life, and one of the richest sources of bioavailable silicon you can find anywhere. It boasts an amazing 15 minerals and is a good source of bioflavonoids too. Drink horsetail tea as much as three times a day.

Remember, it may have taken years for your body to become depleted in essential minerals and trace elements. A few weeks of herbal help is not so long to wait to restore your nails, hair and skin to a healthy balance.

horsetail tea

▶ *2 tsp dried horsetail*
▶ *1 cup boiling water*

Put the dried plant in a tea pot. Pour the boiling water over it and allow it to infuse for 15-20 minutes. Strain, and drink.

▶ dutch rush, a relative of horsetail

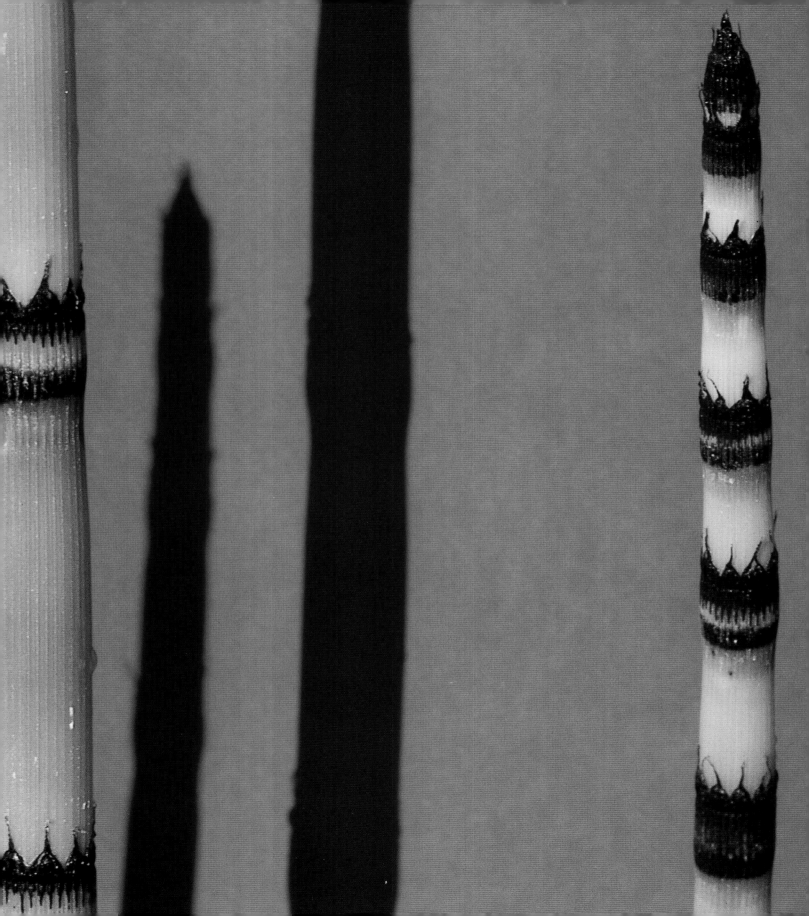

get the essentials

When your body is deficient in essential fatty acids – and this happens often in people who eat a diet high in processed foods – the skin's cell membranes, which are vital for good retention of moisture, become weakened and damaged. Your skin then becomes progressively drier and highly prone to wrinkling and sagging. Udo's Choice (see Resources) is a perfect balance of both Omega 3 and Omega 6 essential fatty acids. Taking 2 tablespoons of it every day provides your body with a perfect supply. You can use it to dress salads or pour it over baked potatoes or cooked vegetables, but never heat it or it loses its goodness completely.

Another fatty acid that is particularly helpful to skin health and good looks is gamma linolenic acid (GLA). You will find it in the seeds of borage, starflower or evening primrose plants. Try taking two 500 mg capsules of one of these oils with each meal.

Proper elimination is also vital to the health of your skin. Constipation ruins good looks – check out page 199 for herb help, and make sure you drink plenty of clean water – spring or filtered. It helps detoxify the skin, dissolving hard debris that interferes with proper circulation and the efficient removal of wastes.

slow down damage

Central to the ageing of skin is the disruption of DNA in its cells caused by free-radical damage. A free-radical is a molecule with an unpaired electron searching for a mate. It can cause chain reactions by reacting with other molecules, destroying cell membranes, damaging DNA and wreaking havoc with the body. This results in degenerative changes to collagen and elastin – the structures that keep the skin firm and elastic. You end up with sagging, wrinkled skin. Many things cause the production of free radicals – sunlight, stress, air pollution, pesticides in foods, cigarette smoke, even excessive exercise. A well-nourished, healthy body is equipped to handle them. But when too many free-radicals are produced in your system, as they often are in modern urban life, you need extra antioxidant help to quench them. So look to vitamins A, C, E, and especially plants replete with antioxidants (see overleaf), including herbs like

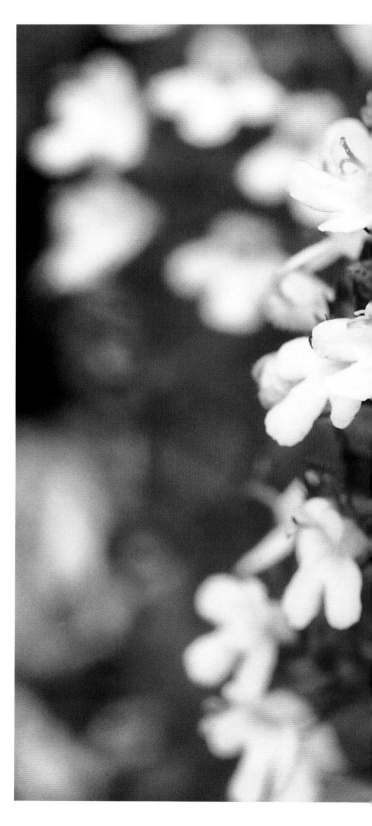

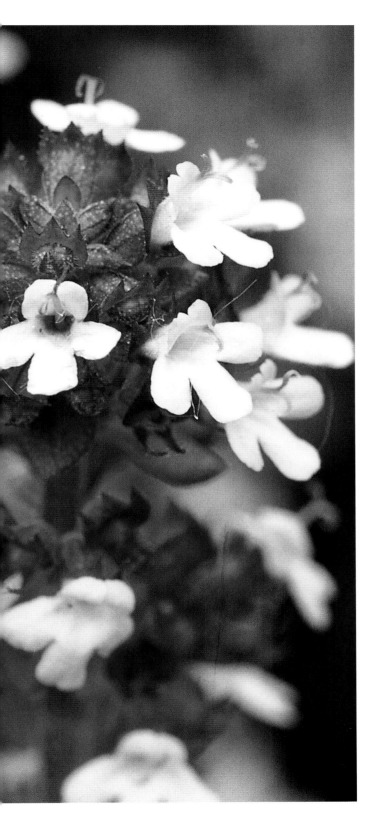

rosemary, lemon balm, horse chestnut, peppermint, thyme and sage. Try my antioxidant tea (overleaf) and include lots of fresh leaves in your salads, such as spinach, rocket, chicory and dandelion.

Vitamin C and the bioflavonoids found in natural foods (such as the whitish inner skin of grapefruit) keep skin young by helping to protect the collagen fibres and keep them intact. So try to include some of these foods in your diet too. Flavonoids (see overleaf) help to ensure the health of the tiny capillaries that supply nutrients to the skin's cells, protecting skin from fragile or broken veins and early wrinkling. When capillaries are not strong and healthy then the skin's cells don't receive all the oxygen and nutrients they need via the bloodstream and their functioning suffers and wastes are not properly eliminated. This is a major contribution to cellulite.

I have a secret weapon against ageing. I keep a bottle of it in my fridge and take it with me wherever I travel. It's a potent mixture of tinctures packed full of skin helpers that includes plenty of vitamin C, strengthening minerals and protective antioxidants.

Echinacea, too, is invaluable to skin as it not only helps maintain good collagen and elastin, it also protects against the breakdown of hyaluronic acid. Hyaluronic acid is the intercellular cement that forms a barrier against infection and helps keep skin strong, resilient and youthful. As the body ages, hyaluronic acid is attacked by an enzyme so that it loses its viscosity and changes from a firm jelly to a thin, watery fluid. Echinacea protects skin from breakdown by blocking the activity of the destructive enzyme.

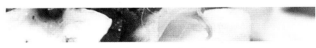

anti-ageing herbal formula

▶ *tincture of echinacea*
▶ *tincture of elderberry*
▶ *tincture of horsetail*

Into a bottle pour equal quantities of the tinctures. Take 1 teaspoon of the mixture in a little water three times a day.

◀ thyme

from inside out

Nutrient	What it does	Where you find it
Vitamin A	A deficiency can cause dry, scaly skin, enlarged pores and acne. Vitamin A is a powerful antioxidant.	◆ Eat plenty of carrots. Eat liver twice a week, or supplement with 10,000 iu of Vitamin A each day. Use burdock, flax seeds, self-heal, chickweed, dandelion, nettle, parsley and watercress as often as possible.
B Complex Vitamins	A deficiency can result in redness, tenderness or ulceration around the mouth, and premature colourloss from hair.	◆ Eat liver twice a week. Or take a tablespoonful of unsulphured black molasses in fruit juice, porridge or yoghurt every day. Use seaweeds liberally in your salads and soups. Add burdock, flax seeds, self-heal, chickweed, comfrey, dandelion and nettle to your diet.
Vitamin C	A deficiency can result in broken veins and premature sagging and wrinkling of the skin. Vitamin C is a powerful antioxidant.	◆ Use elderberry – one of the richest sources of vitamin C. You can take ½ teaspoon tincture of elderberry three times a day. Supplement with 1-2 g vitamin C a day with meals. Vitamin C is also found in borage, self-heal, chickweed, dandelion and nettle. You don't need to worry about taking too much vitamin C. Your body simply flushes out any it doesn't need.
Flavonoids	Flavonoids help absorption of vitamin C in the body and are important for the manufacture of new collagen and elastin in skin.	◆ Flavonoids are found in plants with a high vitamin C content such as elderberries, in the white inner skin of grapefruit, in yellow and orange fruits and vegetables, also in garlic, and in herbs such as yarrow, marshmallow, burdock, calendula, camomile, meadowsweet, hops, St John's wort, mint, self-heal, sage and thyme.
Vitamin E	A deficiency can result in dry, rough, etched or tired-looking skin. Vitamin E is another powerful antioxidant.	◆ Add wheatgerm oil to your diet. Take flax seeds with your breakfast (see the Herbal Cleanse on pages 40-7). Eat a handful of sunflower seeds every day. Supplement with 400 iu vitamin E a day. Caution: vitamin E should be taken only in lower doses if you have a tendency to high blood pressure.
Essential fatty acids	A deficiency of essential fatty acids means the cell membranes vital for good retention of moisture become weakened and damaged and skin becomes progressively drier.	◆ Use Udo's Choice (see Resources): pour 2 tablespoons a day over your salads and cooked vegetables. Supplement with evening primrose, borage or starflower oil. Take 1-2 capsules (500 mg) with each meal.

Nutrient	What it does	Where you find it
Silicon	A deficiency can lead to brittle hair and nails and prematurely ageing skin.	◆ Drink organic horsetail tea (see page 132) three times a day or take ½ – 1 teaspoon tincture of horsetail three times a day.
Zinc	A deficiency can show up in slow-to-heal skin, blemishes, stretch marks and lifeless hair.	◆ Supplement with 25 mg of zinc citrate or picolinate once a day. Eat pumpkin seeds or pine kernels.
Sulphur	A deficiency can result in weakened hair and nails and scaly skin.	◆ Eat a few organic eggs a week, and plenty of garlic.
Selenium	A deficiency can result in poor skin elasticity and early ageing.	◆ Eat plenty of organic eggs, garlic, tuna fish and onion.
Iron	A deficiency can result in dull and lifeless hair and brittle nails.	◆ Use seaweeds liberally in salads and soups. Take a tablespoonful of unsulphured black molasses in fruit juice, porridge or yoghurt every day.
Iodine	A deficiency can lead to lank and lifeless hair and a poorly functioning thyroid.	◆ Use seaweeds liberally in salads and soups. Eat plenty of parsley.
Magnesium	A deficiency can cause dull and lifeless hair and brittle nails.	◆ Drink dandelion tea three times a day (see page 44). Take a tablespoonful of unsulphured organic black molasses in fruit juice, porridge or yoghurt every day.
Potassium	A deficiency can cause dull and lifeless hair and brittle nails.	◆ Eat lots of organic fresh green vegetables each day.
Antioxidants	Antioxidants help prevent free-radical damage, which leads to premature ageing.	◆ Make use of ginseng, ginger and garlic, or drink two cups of antioxidant tea a day – use a mixture of rosemary, lemon balm, peppermint, thyme and sage.

slip into sleep

That old chestnut 'I need my beauty
sleep' happens to be true ...

It is while you are peacefully letting go that your body is busily repairing the damage the day has done. Your skin regenerates and rejuvenates during sleep. When you haven't had enough sleep your face will let you know about it as soon as you look in the mirror next morning – dull eyes, lips and complexion. Deep, regular sleep can do more to enhance your good looks than the most expensive creams and potions on the market.

how long, how deep

There are no hard and fast rules about how much sleep you should get. Some people need a full eight hours. Others thrive on six or even five. The better your diet – the higher it is in fresh fruits, vegetables and unprocessed foods – and the more exercise you get daily, the less time you are likely to need for sleep. What really matters is the quality of your sleep. Sleeping deeply does not mean drugging yourself into oblivion. In Britain alone, 50 million sleeping pills are swallowed each year. These drugs suppress vital rapid-eye-movement or REM phases of sleep, which in turn can produce psychological repression. Herbs offer a far safer alternative, and bring no side-effects or morning 'hangover'.

There are three medically recognized types of insomnia – transient, acute and chronic. Transient insomnia lasts from a few days to a few weeks. It is usually linked to something specific – a worrying event or an illness. In acute insomnia your body has learned poor sleep patterns over a month or more and just keeps repeating them over and over again. Both these types of insomnia can be greatly helped by herbs. Chronic insomnia – when it has lasted more than six months – needs more help than short-term remedies can supply. The underlying reason for your inability to slumber peacefully – be it physical or emotional – needs to be identified and addressed.

nature's tranquillizer

The drug Valium takes its name from a plant: valerian (*Valeriana officinalis*). This was the primary herbal sedative used on both sides of the Atlantic before the advent of barbiturate sleeping pills. It is a safe and well-tested herbal remedy with a smell like dirty old socks. But don't let that put you off since valerian is a powerful herb for inducing safe sleep – more potent than hops or camomile.

You can take valerian in a couple of ways. I like the tincture best. Drink 10 to 20 drops in a little water before bedtime or in the middle of the night when you awaken. Alternatively, take a couple of capsules of the dried root.

Valerian in lower doses is equally useful when your nerves feel 'shot', even during the day. Remarkably, it can enhance your ability to deal with stress and bring you stamina while it calms. Very occasionally, and only to a very few people, valerian will cause a hangover in the morning, if this happens, lower the dose or try a different herb.

powerful passiflora

Passionflower (*Passiflora incarnata*) is a climbing plant with extraordinarily beautiful flowers. It also has a blissful sedative effect on the body. Passionflower is most useful if you wrestle with nervous tension. It can be particularly helpful to women around the time of menopause.

Not as strong as valerian in its actions, passiflora is more calming than sedating. As such, it is a great alternative to tranquillizing drugs. But it is my own personal favourite for sleep. I even like the taste. Use 10-20 drops of the tincture in water or take two capsules of the dried extract up to four times a day when you need it, or make an infusion (see page 126). As an anti-stress herb, passionflower it taken by many people throughout the day in small doses to calm nerves and consequently make everything easier to cope with.

seek sanctuary

Create a sleep sanctuary – somewhere you will enjoy going to rest and sleep. Don't have a television in the room and as far as possible avoid noise and light disturbance. If you awaken in the night, don't turn on the lights. Research has shown that 15 minutes of light in the night can affect levels of melatonin in the body and make it difficult to get back to sleep.

camomile calms

The Latin name *Matricaria camomilla* is derived either from mater meaning mother, or from *matrix* meaning womb. It has been used for thousands of years to calm anxiety and induce sleep. The easiest way to take camomile is as a tea (see page 47) before bed or whenever you need relaxation. Camomile also works well as a relaxant and sleep enhancer when taken together with passionflower.

relaxing hops

You can use the flowers from the hop plant (*Humulus lupulus*) together with other remedies as a treatment for everything from indigestion to agitated nerves. Like valerian, hops have a pronounced sedative effect but it is a far milder remedy.

Unlike valerian, hops smell sweet and you can use them without worrying about possible side-effects. You can take hops in the form of a tincture too. But by far the best way for sleep – particularly good for people who awaken in the middle of the night and have trouble going back to sleep – is to drink hop tea (see page 125). Put the tea – sweetened with honey if you like – by the side of your bed so that you can drink it should you awaken in the night. It is also a good idea to use a little pillow stuffed with dried hop blossoms. Put it under your neck when you go to bed or if ever you awaken at night.

sleep enhancers

make a sleep pillow

Herb pillows are small cushions filled with fragrant, sleep-inducing herbs, that you can tuck under your normal pillow or keep near you while you sleep. Once you have stuffed your pillow don't sew it up too tightly so you can replace the herbs as often as you wish. If you keep it inside another pillowcase you will easily keep it clean.

Herbs for relaxation include camomile, thyme, lavender, catmint and rosemary, but my favourite pillows include a high proportion of dried hops. A few drops of essential oil of camomile will help with sleeplessness, geranium will relieve anxiety and lavender irritation. Sprinkling with a little orris root powder will help preserve the mixture but this can cause allergic reactions in some people (see page 93).

socks with a difference

This is a sure-fire help for sleeplessness. It was taught to me by a wonderful medical doctor, Philip Kilsby. The trouble is that when I tell people about it they often think I'm joking. But you will never know how well it works until you try it.

Wet a pair of cotton socks in cold water and wring them out so that they are no longer dripping. Put them on and then cover them with a pair of dry woollen socks, then pop into bed. Leave the socks on for at least half an hour, although it doesn't matter if they stay on all night should you fall asleep.

face the world

What is the point of making your own cosmetics when you can walk into a shop and buy some very nice ones? ...

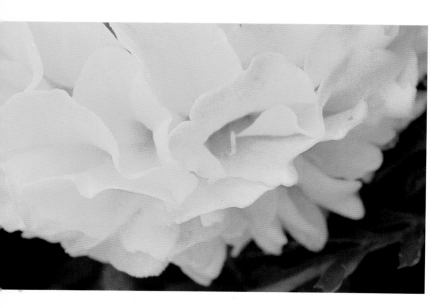

The reasons are freshness and fun. Herbs work wonders on skin, which is why they find their way into so many commercial preparations. But they work best when they are fresh. Manufacturers of shop-bought cosmetics have to use chemical stabilizers and preservatives simply because they don't know how long the product is going to have to stay on the shelf – both in the shop and in your bathroom. By creating your own cleansers, toners and moisturizers you are able to regularly make small amounts from the freshest ingredients – and nothing is better for your skin. The more often you make them the better you will be at adjusting the ingredients so they suit your skin to perfection, and your skin will never get tired of them.

where do I start?

Home-made cosmetics are simple to make. And it's much cheaper to make mistakes than when you are buying them. With so many herbs to choose from you will never be at a loss for something new to try. I have listed a few herbs that are good for certain skin types, but this is by no means an exclusive list. To keep things simple the herb infusions included in the recipes for skin care below and overleaf are made to the same proportions – 4 teaspoons of dried herb (or 7-8 of fresh) to a cup of boiling water. As you become more familiar with the recipes you can make your infusions stronger or weaker. Don't be afraid to experiment with the herbs and the recipes. And remember to alter your formulas to allow for what your skin needs as the seasons change.

herbal cleanser

The perfect cleanser caresses your face with the gentlest touch as it erases the day's dirt from your skin. You can't go far wrong by starting with an oil and honey cleansing base. The honey soothes while the oil dissolves the

herbal cleanser

▶ *8 tsp your choice of fresh herb or 4 tsp dried*
▶ *1 cup boiling water*
▶ *1 tsp of almond, apricot or grapeseed oil*
▶ *1 tsp good quality honey*

Make a herb infusion by putting the fresh or dried herb into a tea pot and pouring the boiling water over it. Allow to steep for 10-15 minutes. While your infusion is steeping, put the oil and honey into a small bowl and warm it gently over hot water until the honey dissolves. Add 2 teaspoons of the infusion and mix well.

choosing your herbs

herbs to brighten dry skin	herbs to soothe sensitive skin	herbs to calm oily skin
◆ Camomile, comfrey leaf and root, dandelion, elderflower, fennel, liquorice, mint, orris root, parsley, yarrow.	◆ Calendula, comfrey, cranberry, elderflower, figwort, lavender, rose, yarrow.	◆ Elderflower, lady's mantle, lavender, lemon grass, liquorice, mint, rose, rosemary, sage, witch hazel.

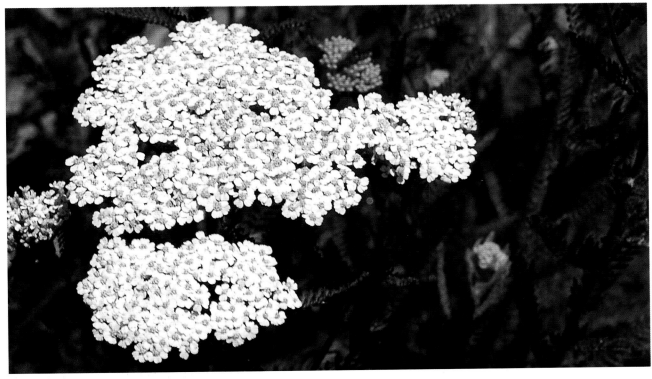

◄ calendula ▲ yarrow

grease and grime of the day. Work it well into your face with clean fingers and rinse off with warm water. Make this lotion fresh every day if you can – it really doesn't keep more than a couple of days.

refresher course

Toners stimulate and refresh the skin. Use them after cleansing, after a face mask, or put some in a plant spray and spritz your face with it whenever you need to freshen up.

If your skin is sensitive, simply make an infusion as if you were making a cleansing lotion (using 4 teaspoons of dried herb to 1 cup of water), cool it, put it in the fridge and apply it with cotton wool after cleansing. Camomile, yarrow, sage, mint, fennel and lady's mantle are all excellent astringent herbs.

For less sensitive skin make a stronger cup of infusion and add a teaspoon of cider vinegar. For oily skin, add a teaspoon of lemon juice and a teaspoon of witch hazel to your infusion. The cider vinegar and lemon juice will restore your skin's natural (slightly acid) pH.

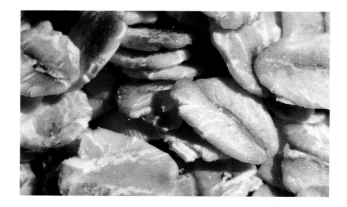

mighty moisturizer

▶ *2 tsp beeswax*
▶ *2 tsp cocoa butter (or if you are really stuck, creamed coconut)*
▶ *3 tbsp almond, apricot or grapeseed oil*
▶ *1 tbsp spring or rose water*
▶ *½ tbs of aloe vera gel*
▶ *2 tbsp of herb infusion (see cleansing lotion, page 140): choose from: calendula, comfrey, rose, elderflower, marshmallow or yarrow*
▶ *capsule vitamin E*
▶ *a few drops of your favourite essential oil (optional)*

Put the beeswax, cocoa butter and almond/apricot or grapeseed oil into a double boiler and warm over a low heat until the beeswax has melted. Let the mixture cool slightly.

Add your aloe vera gel and herbal infusion to the water and put it in a blender and – much as you would make mayonnaise – blend in the oil mixture drop by drop so it emulsifies. Blend until the cream is white and thick. Squeeze in the capsule of vitamin E and add your essential oil if this is what you have chosen. Put your cream into jars and keep it in the fridge.

Note: If you have difficulty making the oil and water mix and you find it continually curdles, try adding 2 tablespoons of liquid lecithin to the distilled water and

lazy oatmeal mask

▶ *2 tbsp herb infusion (see page 140)*
▶ *2 tbsp natural yoghurt*
▶ *finely ground oatmeal*

Put the herb infusion and natural yoghurt in a bowl and then slowly add the finely ground oatmeal until you have a workable paste. Put it all over your face and neck, nice and thick. Relax for 10 minutes and then wash off with plenty of warm water. This is another wonderful mask to use in the bath. When you have washed it off your face the oatmeal goes on working in the bath to soften the rest of your skin with no extra effort from you at all.

preventing drought

It may take some trial and error to create the perfect moisturizer, but it's well worth it (and fun). To the left is a simple water-in-oil emulsion, which works for both dry and oily skins. Make your moisturizer in small quantities and note down any changes you make to the proportions. Apply it twice a day under make-up or on its own.

holiday treats

Give your skin a break and treat it to some luxurious pampering. Your skin will thank you. Do this by turning a herb infusion into a face mask (see left).

deep steam

A facial sauna can deep cleanse and stimulate skin. Begin by thoroughly cleansing your skin. Take 2 handfuls of fresh herbs or 2 tablespoons of dried and put them in a bowl. You can use wonderfully refreshing herbs such as nettle that you otherwise might hesitate to put on your skin. Cover with hot water and lean your head over the bowl, placing a towel over your head to keep the steam in. Steam for 5 minutes. Use a toner afterwards to close the pores, or splash with cool water. Choose from borage, calendula, camomile, comfrey, elderflowers, lavender, nettle, rosemary, sage and yarrow.

Caution:
if you have thread veins or are prone to flushing, don't use a facial steam.

▲ whole oats   ▶ aloe vera

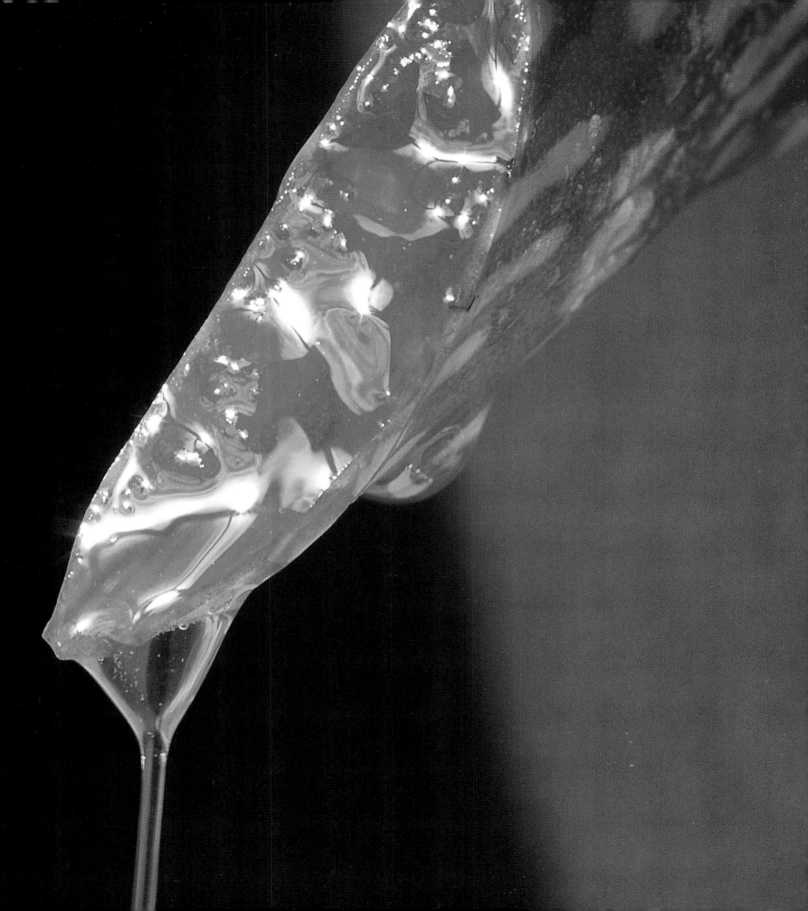

caring hands

Gone are the glorious 1940s and 1950s when no self-respecting lady left the house without a pair of gloves. No gentleman would be seen driving his car ungloved either. Now we just thrust our hands in our pockets or leave them hanging around in dry winds, burning sun, or piercing cold. Take time out to care for your hands. It is a great way to relax all over. There are few jobs you can be getting on with if your hands are busy being pampered.

daily duty

Daily moisturizing is just as important for hands as faces. After all, they are exposed to the outside world in just the same way. Use the recipe given below, but if you do nothing else, rub a little of your facial moisturizer over your hands when you apply it to your face. But don't miss out on this delicious hand lotion.

You can make a basic unperfumed cream base into something really special by adding a herbal infusion. There are some very good cream bases that you can buy (see Resources), or you can use the recipe given below to make your own. You can add up to a quarter of the cream's weight in herb infusion to make sweet scented and nourishing hand creams.

Adding an extract rather than an infusion will make the cream even more potent. I particularly like calendula, lavender, elderflower and sage infusions (4 teaspoons of the dried herb infused in a cup of hot water for 10 minutes), or adding a little rose water.

hand lotion

► *3 tbsp glycerine*
► *1 tsp arrowroot powder*
► *4 tsp dried herb of your choice (see below)*

Put the glycerine into a bowl and add the arrowroot powder. Mix well. You can now add 1 tablespoon of a herbal infusion made by steeping the dried herb of your choice in a cup of hot water for 10 minutes. Mix the infusion into the glycerine mixture well and decant the lotion into a beautiful bottle. Use it daily to soften and beautify your hands.
Choose your infusion from:
► lavender for delicious scent
► camomile or elderflower for softening
► marshmallow for soothing
► fresh rose petals for their rejuvenating reputation. If you decide on rose, you can add a little extra style by slipping a teaspoon of rose water into your lotion.

cream base

► *2 tsp beeswax*
► *2 tsp coconut oil (or creamed coconut if you are really stuck)*
► *3 tbsp almond, apricot or grapeseed oil*
► *1 tbsp aloe vera gel (buy pure aloe vera gel rather than using your own plant)*
► *2 tbsp water*

Put the beeswax, coconut oil and almond, apricot, or grapeseed oil into a double boiler and warm over a low heat until the beeswax has melted. Let the mixture stand for a little. Mix the aloe vera gel and the water in a blender and – much as you would make mayonnaise – blend in the oil mixture drop by drop so it emulsifies. Blend until the cream is white and thick. Put into jars and keep in the fridge until you are ready to use them.

hot oil – for hands too

Just as you give your hair an occasional intensive treatment to soften and condition, you can give extra-dry hands conditioning help too. On page 197 you will find my emergency 'gardener's hands' overnight cleaning and softening treatment for when your skin is very bad. For less desperate situations use a hot oil treatment, as outlined below. You can use olive oil, or almond oil if you find olive oil a little too heavy.

tough as nails

There's nothing that works quite so well to strengthen and condition your nails as drinking horsetail tea every day (see page 132). It is full of minerals – most importantly silica – which the body needs to build strong nails and hair. Adding seaweeds to your soups and salads daily will also do a great deal to create beautiful nails and hair. You can improve the look of your nails and encourage strong growth by giving your cuticles a treat at least once a week. This is best done after soaking your hands in a hand bath, when the cuticles are soft and pliable. If you have long neglected your nails, rub the oil into your cuticles every day for a few weeks.

hand bathing

Give your hands the equivalent of a long, relaxing soak in the bath. Find a bowl or tub that is big enough for you to rest your hands in comfortably for 15 minutes at a time and use the same herbs you would use to nourish your skin in the bath such as camomile or comfrey. Either put them straight into the bowl or dangle them in the water in a bath bag. My personal favourite formulas for hand bathing (and bath bathing) are camomile smoothie and comfrey brightener (see below). Pour enough comfortably hot water over your herbs to cover your hands. Swish the loose herbs or bath bag around, dip your hands in, and relax. After 10-15 minutes take your hands out and gently pat them dry with a warm towel.

hot oil treatment

▶ *1 tbsp olive or almond oil*
▶ *5 drops favourite essential oil or 3 tsp dried sage*

Warm the olive or almond oil over hot water and add either the essential oil drops or 1 teaspoon of strong sage infusion (3 teaspoons of dried sage steeped in a cup of warm water for 10 minutes). Mix well. Start to work the oil into your hands, beginning with the tips of your fingers and working back towards the wrists. Give your skin a good massage for at least 5 minutes to help circulation. Wash the oil off with warm water and a little mild soap. Then pat your hands dry with a warm towel.

cuticle nourishment

▶ *1 tbsp almond oil*
▶ *2 drops essential oil of lavender*

Take the almond oil and add the essential oil. Keep in a bottle in the fridge. After soaking your hands, gently push your cuticles back with an orange stick. Rub a little of the oil over your nails and into your cuticles and massage well.

hand baths

Camomile smoothie:
Into a bath bag put equal quantities of camomile, elderflowers, comfrey and linden blossoms.

Comfrey brightener:
Into a bath bag put equal quantities of comfrey, nettle, dandelion and orange peel.

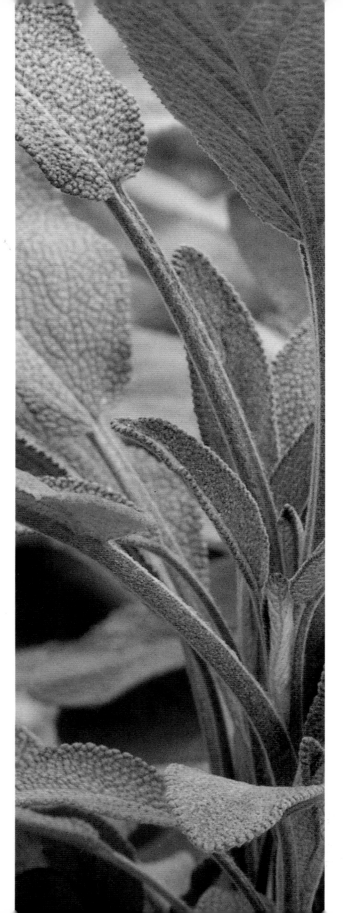

hair raising

Your hair is a terrible give-away ...

Whenever you eat badly, over-work or are generally run-down, your hair dulls and loses its bounce quicker than a puppy wanting a walk. Treat it well on the outside. Use gentle herb shampoos to preserve its natural oils, rinses to restore its pH balance and the occasional conditioning treatment to nourish and smooth. As long as you treat your hair well in this way it will be less likely to snitch on the occasional lapse of lifestyle.

wash and go

You can create a herbal shampoo in two ways. Make your own shampoo base using pure soap to which you add a herbal infusion, or buy a mild shampoo and add your infusion. I prefer to buy the mildest shampoo I can find since I find pure soap doesn't really suit my hair. It leaves it a bit dull even when I use plenty of herb rinses. Try both shampoo bases (given below and opposite bottom) for yourself. It's an inexpensive and fun way to find out what your hair likes best.

pure soap shampoo base

▶ *50 g (2 oz) soap flakes*
▶ *600 ml (1 pint) warm water*

Add the flakes to the warm water and allow them to dissolve. Keep your shampoo base in an attractive jar in the bathroom (if you put it in any old jam jar I can guarantee you won't use it). It should make enough for five good shampoos.

◀ sage, ▲ comfrey

146

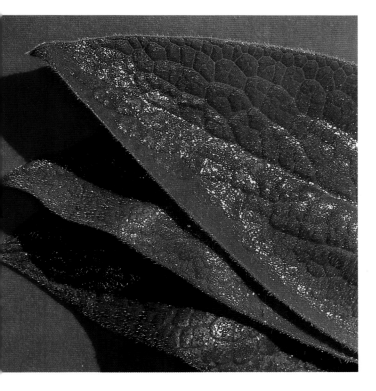

shampooing herbs

hair type	herbs
Normal	◆ Lavender, rose, rosemary.
Dry	◆ Calendula, elderflower, marshmallow, nettle. Add a teaspoon of almond or apricot oil to your shampoo and mix together well.
Greasy	◆ Burdock, calendula, elderflower, horsetail, lemon balm, mint, sage, yarrow.
Damaged	◆ Calendula, comfrey, lavender.
Thinning	◆ Nettle, parsley, peppermint.
Dandruff	◆ Artichoke leaves, burdock, cleavers, comfrey, nettle, rosemary, sage, willow bark.
Dull	◆ Horsetail, nettle, rosemary, sage.
Fly away	◆ Calendula. Add a beaten egg to your shampoo.

Make your shampoo fresh every time you wash your hair. In this way your infusion will not have 'gone off' between shampoos, and you can use a different herbal infusion when you want to. Take a few minutes to massage half of the shampoo into your scalp. Rinse, and use the rest of the shampoo all over your hair. Rinse with plenty of warm water.

dilute shampoo base

▶ *mild shampoo*
▶ *water*

Find a mild shampoo that you like. Go along the chemist's shelves comparing the ingredients on the bottles until you find the one with as few chemical ingredients as possible. Once home, dilute it by half. The easiest way to do this is to pour the shampoo into a bowl, refill the bottle with warm water, and mix it into the shampoo. Keep this base in an attractive jar in the bathroom.

shampoo herbal infusion

▶ *6 tbsp fresh herb or 3 tbsp dried*
▶ *½ cup boiling water*
▶ *essential oil (optional)*

Make a strong infusion by putting the herbs into a tea pot and pouring the water over the top. Allow to steep for 10 minutes. Make sure it has cooled, then strain and add 1 tablespoon of infusion to 4 tablespoons of the soap base. You can also add a couple of drops of essential oil for fragrance.

rinse and refresh

Following your shampoo with a herb rinse will help to restore the natural, slightly acid pH of healthy hair. It will also make your hair shine, and with the right herbs it will bring out its natural colour and highlights (see the chart opposite). You can use lemon juice or cider vinegar, whatever you have to hand. Lemon juice is particularly good if you have fair hair.

hot oil conditioner

Give your hair an occasional conditioning treatment if it is dry or damaged. Apply your oil and essential oil mixture and mix evenly over your scalp (not your hair) and massage well. If you have long hair, pin it up loosely all over your head. Soak a towel in hot water and ring it out. Wrap your head in the hot towel and cover with a shower cap or tin foil. Sit back and relax for an hour.

For some real relaxation, soak another towel in hot water, wring it out well and place it over your face. You will find that it does wonders to revive all those tired facial muscles. Use a herb shampoo to wash the oil out (don't wet your hair before applying the shampoo). Then rinse with plenty of warm water.

tropical treat

Coconut oil makes a sublime conditioner for dry hair. You can buy it very cheaply by the jar from health-food stores and chemists. Put 2 teaspoons of coconut oil in a small bowl over warm water. As it begins to soften, add 2-3 drops of your favourite essential oil – try rosemary, bergamot, lavender, geranium, or ylang ylang. Mix the essence in well.

Now massage the softened oil into your scalp and smooth it along the hair shafts. Put the oil back in the bowl to warm it if it starts to go hard again. Pile your hair on top of your head and cover with a small (dry) warm towel and a shower cap to stop the oil getting all over the furniture. Leave it on for an hour. Then shampoo the oil out using your usual herbal shampoo (don't wet your hair first) and rinse with plenty of warm water. You will need two to three 'soapings' to clear all the oil.

rinse recipe

▶ 3 tbsp dried herb
▶ ½ cup water
▶ 1 tbsp lemon juice or cider vinegar
▶ 600 ml (1 pint) warm water

Make an infusion by steeping the dried herbs in the water, just as you did for the shampoo on the previous page. You can use the same infusion if you wish. Then mix 1 tablespoon of the herb infusion with the lemon juice or cider vinegar and add the warm water.

You will need two large bowls for rinsing, one with the rinse in it and one to catch it. Hold your head over the empty bowl and pour your rinse over it from the other bowl. Repeat this so that you are pouring rinse over your hair from one bowl into the other. Rinse your hair this way three or four times. Leave the final rinse on for a few minutes. Then rinse again with plenty of warm water.

hot oil conditioner

▶ 2 tbsp almond or apricot oil
▶ 2-3 drops essential oil of rosemary, bergamot, lavender, geranium, or tea tree (good for dandruff) or 2 tsp herb infusion

Put the almond or apricot oil into a small bowl and add to it the essential oil and mix in well. Or use 2 teaspoons of a herb infusion, made as for the shampoo or rinse (see left). Stand the bowl in a pan of hot water to allow it to heat a little.

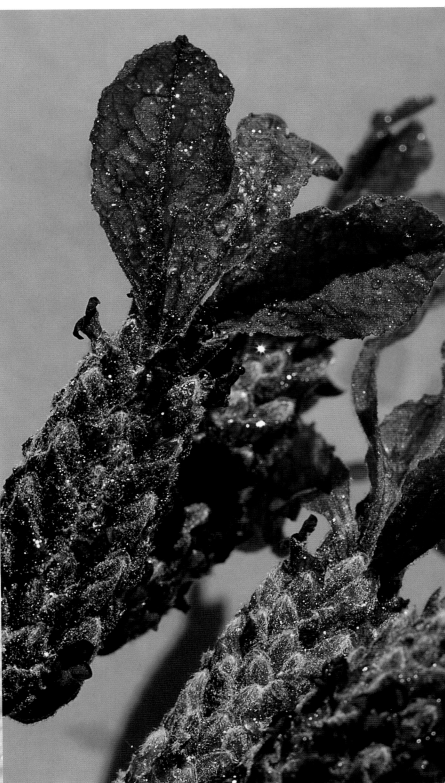

rinsing herbs

hair colour	herbs
Dark	◆ lavender ◆ nettle ◆ rosemary ◆ yarrow
Auburn	◆ calendula ◆ clovel ◆ witch hazel
Brunette	◆ calendula ◆ cloves ◆ lavender ◆ mint ◆ rosemary ◆ sage
Fair	◆ calendula ◆ camomile ◆ mullein
Grey	◆ camomile ◆ rosemary ◆ sage

► rabbit's ear lavender

radiant smiles

A lovely smile can light up your day ...

Bring a gleam to your smile by using fresh and wholesome herbs and you just might find yourself lighting up everyone's day.

tea is for teeth

Green tea (*Camellia sinensis*) has hit the headlines recently for its remarkable antioxidant properties. What you may not have realized is that it does wonderful things for your teeth too. Green tea contains tooth-strengthening soluble fluoride. And on its way through your mouth the tannins it contains help to stop plaque building up around your teeth.

And if you have an irresistable sweet tooth so you always reach for the sugar, help is at hand. Sweeten your tea by adding a little liquorice root to the pot while you are brewing it. Liquorice contains glycyrrhizin, which is antibacterial. It also prevents decay rather than encouraging it as sugar does. For a minty variation, see the recipe on page 57.

clean teeth

You can make your own toothpastes and powders using ingredients you have to hand. Before commercial tooth-pastes, people used many things to clean their teeth, including sea salt. I find this a little too abrasive and have discovered that orris root powder is much kinder yet works just as well (but see page 93). One of the latest fashions in toothpastes has been the addition of bicar-bonate of soda, as it bubbles in your mouth making it feel fresh. You can make your own using ordinary bicar-bonate of soda you would use for cooking.

wash your mouth out

Some commercial mouthwashes are too strong. In fact some can leave you gasping for breath. Instead, rinse out your mouth with a gentle herbal infusion that you make and keep in the fridge (see recipe on page 33). Try a strong peppermint tea for a refreshing rinse.

---

toothsome tea

▶ 1-2 tsp green tea
▶ small piece liquorice root
▶ 1 cup boiling water

Put the green tea in a tea pot with the liquorice root. Then pour the boiling water over it and allow to steep for 5-10 minutes, strain and drink. Slosh it around your mouth well (but don't upset dinner guests).

tooth powder

▶ ½ tsp dried sage
▶ 1 tsp orris root powder
▶ 1-2 drops essential oil of peppermint

Put the dried sage into a mortar with the orris root powder. Pound them together well until you have a powder. Then add the essential oil of peppermint and mix well. Keep your powder in an airt-tight jar and use on a damp toothbrush. Don't swallow it, as any essential oil can be dangerous if ingested. For something a little more zingy, use ½ teaspoon of sage, ¼ teaspoon of orris root powder and ¼ teaspoon of ginger. This really makes your mouth glow.

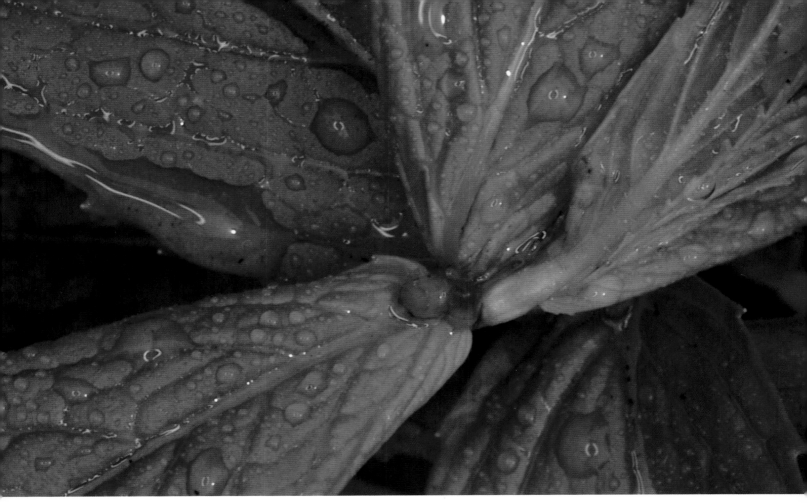

▲ mint

bubbling bicarbonate

▶ *3 tsp sodium bicarbonate*
▶ *3 tsp glycerine*

Put the sodium bicarbonate into a small bowl, add the glycerine and mix well (don't worry, the sodium bicarbonate won't fizz up). Keep it in a jar with a wide enough rim to dip your toothbrush into. You can use this toothpaste just as it is. I don't much like the taste, so I add 3 drops of essential oil – no more than this, as ingesting essential oils can be dangerous. Choose from:
▶ Essential oil of peppermint for its refreshing taste
▶ Essential oil of lavender for breath freshening
▶ Essential oil of myrrh to soothe sore gums.

tipsy teeth

▶ *1 handful fresh herb*
▶ *600 ml (1 pint) white wine*

Crush the herbs slightly and then put into a jar. Add the white wine, seal the jar and leave it in a cool place for a week. Strain and pour into a clean bottle. Use it to rinse your mouth out well and don't worry if you swallow a little – but not too much or you might start your day a little tipsy. Choose your herbs from:
▶ Peppermint – refreshing and tasty
▶ Myrrh – antiseptic and astringent for problem gums
▶ Comfrey – soothing, and full of natural minerals to strengthen teeth.

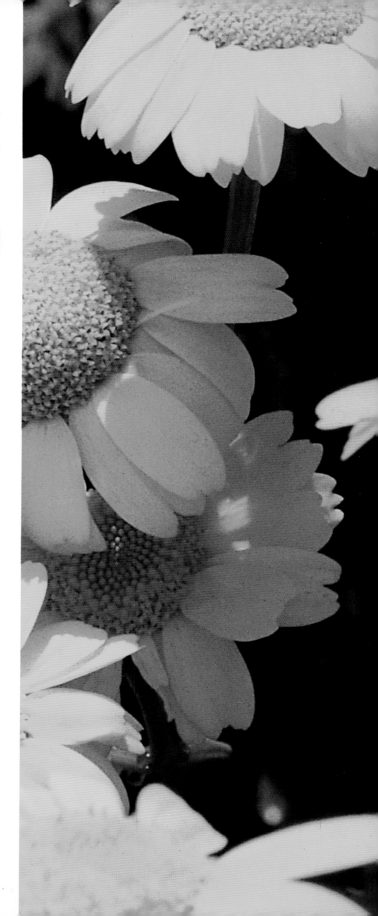

kissable lips

Soft, smooth lips are the frame to a beautiful smile, so make your own healing and soothing lip balm. For fun I melt a little of my favourite lipstick in a bowl over some hot water and add a small amount to the cooling lip balm for just a hint of colour.

luscious lip balm

▶*1 tsp beeswax*
▶*1 tsp coconut oil or cocoa butter*
▶*2 tsp almond or apricot oil*
▶*2 drops essential oil*

Put a teaspoon in the fridge. Put the beeswax, cocoa butter or coconut oil, and apricot or almond oil into a double boiler. Allow the beeswax to melt. To test, take your teaspoon out of the fridge. Dip it into the melted oils and rub a little through your fingers. If it's too runny, add a little more beeswax; too hard, add more almond or apricot oil. When you have a consistency you are happy with, allow it to cool and add your essential oil. Pour into a jar and leave to set. Use whenever your lips feel dry.

lip balm with infused oil

▶*1 handful fresh calendula, camomile or comfrey*
▶*almond or apricot oil*

For added healing and soothing help, infuse a herb in almond or apricot oil. Pack a small glass jar with your fresh herb and pour almond or apricot oil over the herb until the jar is almost full. Put a lid on it and leave in a warm place, preferably on a sunny windowsill, for two to three weeks. Give the jar a good shake daily. Strain the oil through muslin, squeezing out the leaves. Store any left-over oil in a brown glass jar in the refrigerator and mix half St John's wort oil and half plain almond or apricot oil for your First Aid Kit (see page 208).

▶dyer's camomile

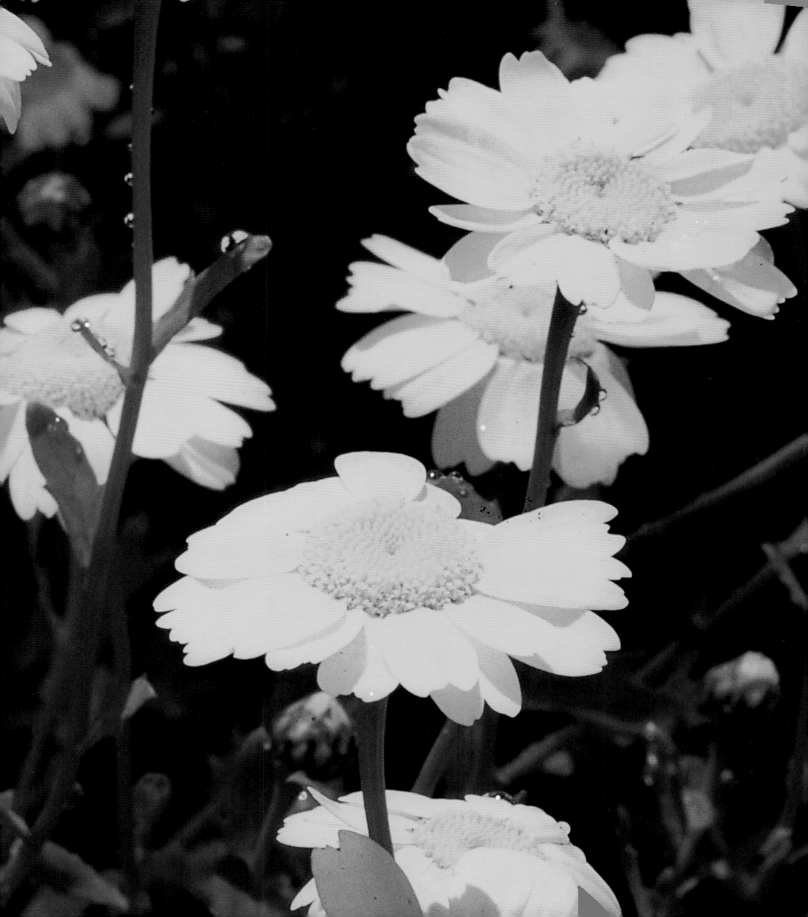

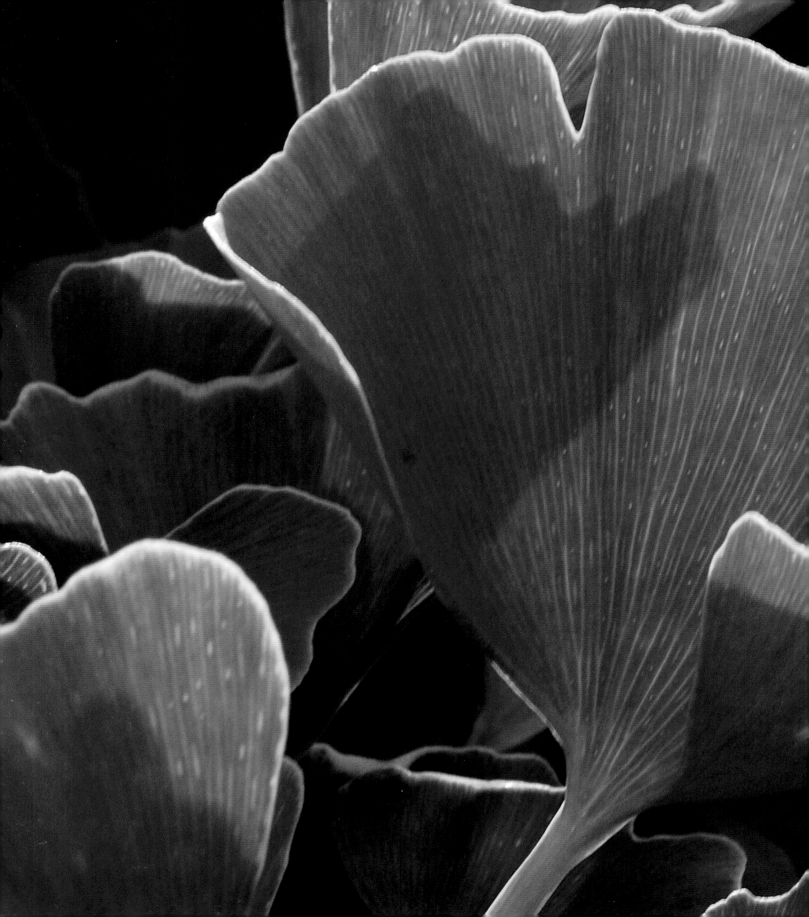

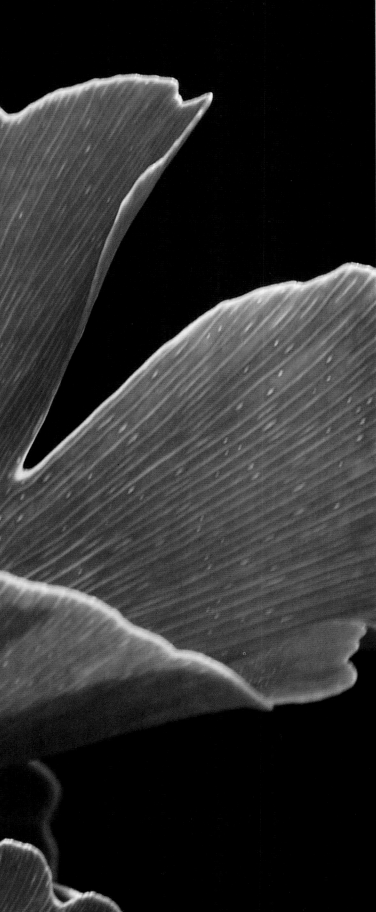

balancing₇

Herbs carry within them an ability to balance what is not in balance in the body in a way that no man-made drug or nutritional supplement can. This makes them our best allies against ageing, our most effective protectors and enhancers for reproduction and the most efficient guardians of our sexual potency. If you have not yet experienced what plants can do for you in these areas of your life, you have some wonderful surprises in store.

◄ gingko

ageless balance

Your biological age does not necessarily have a lot to do with how old you are in years. Herbs can help you stay young – in how you look, how you feel, and the way your body functions. Combined with regular detoxification and a natural diet high in a wide variety of fresh vegetables, they can also rejuvenate your body in medically measurable ways – improved circulation, lowered LDL cholesterol, better use of oxygen and smoother, firmer skin.

Plants rejuvenate in two ways. Some, such as ginseng, garlic and gotu kola, are specifically anti-ageing in their actions. Others – herbs such as purslane and thyme as well as foods like tomatoes, oranges, carrots and green vegetables – are literally brimming with antioxidants and other phytochemicals which are regenerative and immune enhancing. Make these plants an everyday part of your life. They will help protect you from the kind of free-radical damage that underlies both premature ageing and the development of degenerative diseases.

anti-ageing herbs

gotu kola

Centella asiatica has been used for centuries in India to extend lifespan and enhance memory. Gotu kola is easy to grow in your garden or in a pot in the kitchen window. It is also easy to introduce into your life. Just add a fresh leaf or two or a teaspoon of this dried plant to whatever herb tea you are drinking. You can also put a few leaves into salad when you make it.

purslane

Portulaca oleracea brims with antioxidants – both plant chemicals and the vitamins known for their abilities to quench excess free-radicals in the body. It also enhances the immune system. You can grow purslane in a vegetable patch too, or just about anywhere – even in window boxes, between the rose bushes, or wherever you have an extra bit of space. Add purslane to fresh vegetable juices, or put it through a blender to make 'live' vegetable drinks.

ginkgo biloba

This improves circulation to the brain. Lots of well-founded European research now says so. It can even be helpful to people with Alzheimer's disease. The leaves from this most ancient of trees restore memory, elevate mood and quell anxiety. There are more than 300 published studies and reports that support the anti-ageing properties of ginkgo. Its extract is used in Germany to help treat everything from depression and cerebrovascular insufficiency to asthma, transplant rejection and hearing loss. It is also used in expensive skin products to protect against environmental irritation. You can take ginkgo as an extract, tincture, or in capsules. I prefer a high-potency herbal tincture – 1 teaspoon two or three times a day.

Its leaves dazzle. So perfectly shaped are they that they shimmer like thousands of delicate oriental fans waving in the wind. The ginkgo tree is as old as time itself. A simple tree can live for 4,000 years. Little wonder. For the kernels and leaves of this magnificent growing thing are treasure houses of potent anti-ageing antioxidants – so effective that they put vitamin C to shame. The ginkgo is a reassuring tree to lean against too. Its roots tap the earth's deepest sources of healing to draw energy up as a gift to man.

The more than forty studies of *Ginkgo biloba* carried out in the last twenty years confirm that ginkgo leaf increases blood flow all over the body. This helps restore balance in a hundred ways while also countering varicose veins, tinnitus, dizziness, PMS and impotence.

▶ gotu kola

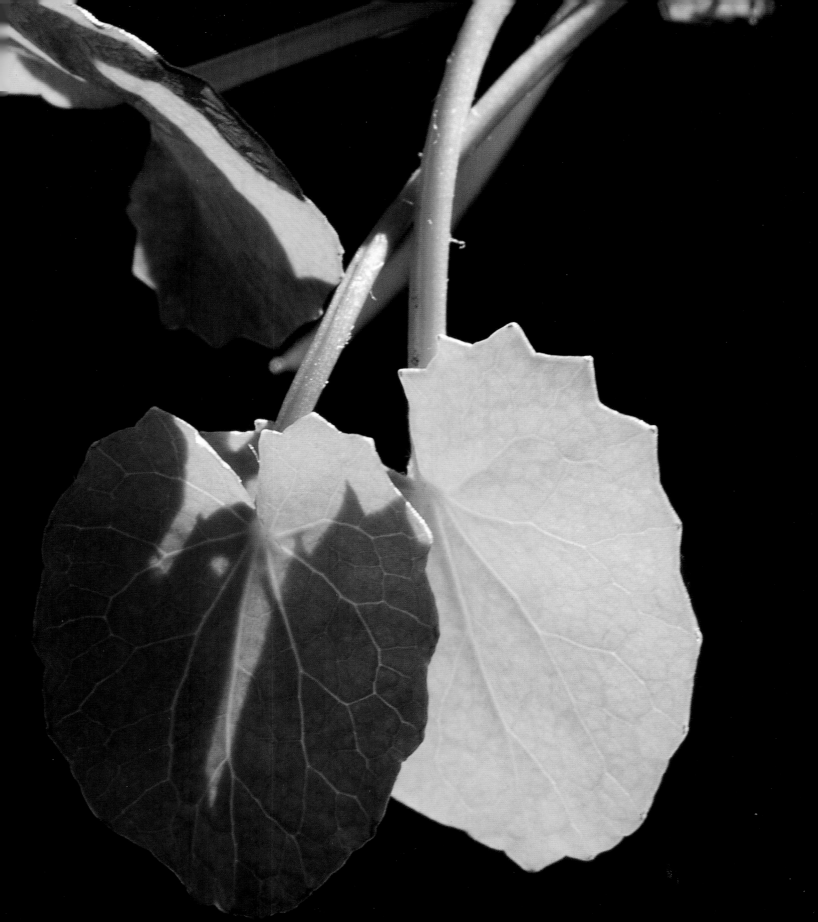

Ginkgo's effect on blood flow to the brain is powerfully anti-ageing. It combats senility, improves Alzheimer-associated dementia, and even aids recovery from stroke. Some 10 million prescriptions a year are written for ginkgo world-wide. The plant's support for memory and attention makes it the herb of choice for the Western high-achiever. Smart people take ginkgo to help make them even smarter and to stay that way. Ginkgo can clear fog from your brain and improve the circulation of energy and oxygen throughout your body.

ginseng

Panax ginseng is the classic anti-ageing plant. It can be a godsend when you are recovering from a long-term illness or stress or pulling yourself out of deep fatigue. And it improves libido in both men and women. This root, which so often looks like a man, brings endurance when you need it. I like to take ginseng as a tea – but make sure you buy a good one (or see page 115). When I need strengthening I drink double doses of ginseng tea that has been specially processed to dissolve instantaneously in hot water (see Resources).

evening primrose

Oenothera biennis boasts seeds rich in essential fatty acids including gamma-linolenic acid – GLA. This oil taken as a supplement in capsule form is enormously helpful to women because of its ability to quell symptoms of PMS, clear dry skin and uplift mood. It mitigates many menopausal problems too. You take it in capsules, 1-2 capsules with meals. Keep them refrigerated, for like all EFAs, GLA oxidizes easily. Also be sure to buy the best quality you can find. You get what you pay for.

horsetail

Horsetail is one of the world's oldest plants. *Equisetum arvense* is the best natural source of the mineral silicon, which declines in the body as we get older. Silicon is important to the maintenance of strong bones, preventing osteoporosis, firming skin and protecting from wrinkles and sagging. You can take it powdered in capsules or purchase silicon derived from horsetail also in capsules. Easier still, drink horsetail tea (see page 132).

► evening primrose

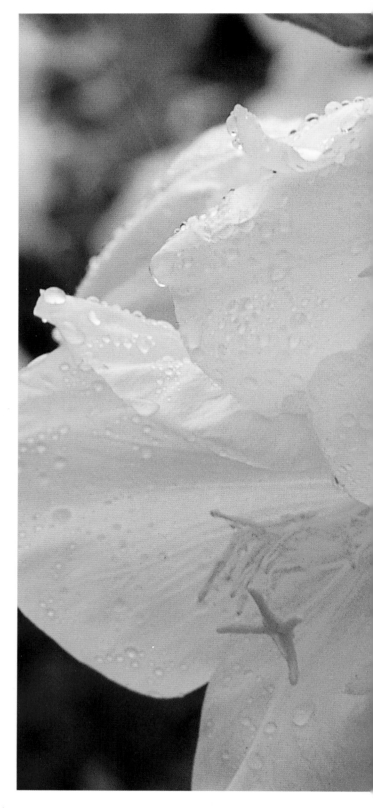

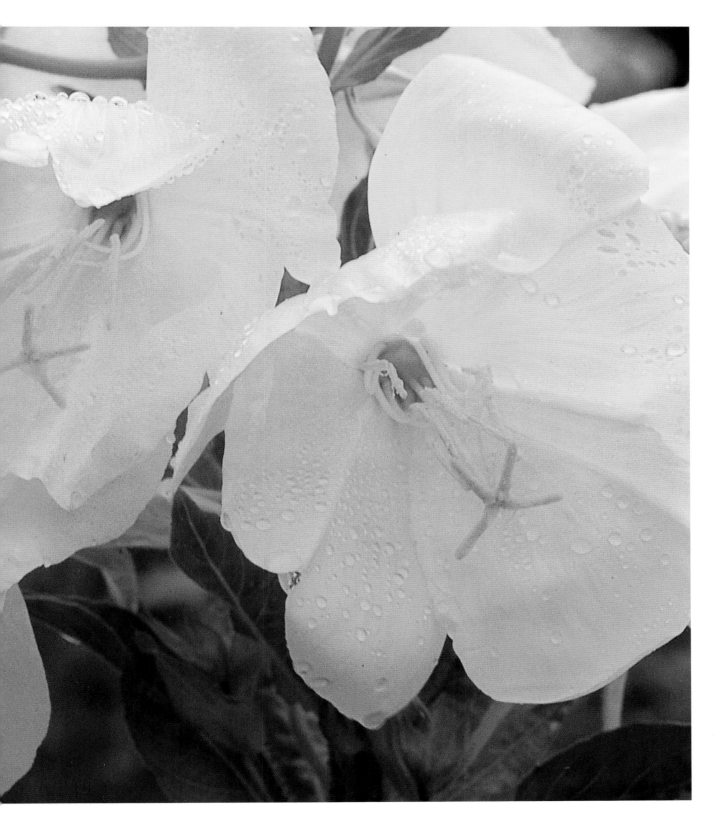

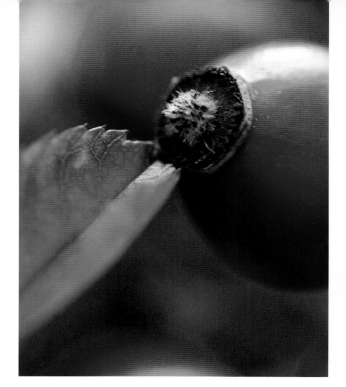

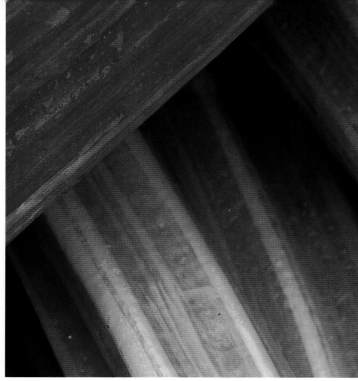

ageless ageing

with phytonutrients ...

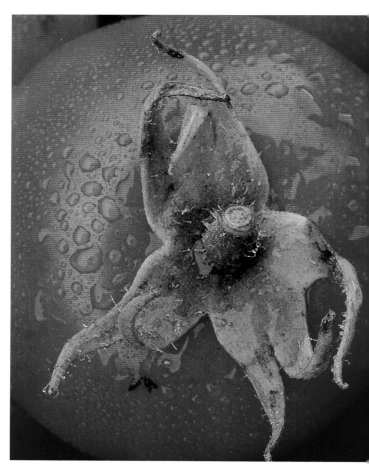

Research into natural chemicals capable of bringing balance to the body and protecting it both from illness and premature ageing is expanding at an exponential rate; and 90% of the best come directly from plants. The list of biologically active plant-based compounds found in herbs, vegetables and fruits, seeds, grains and beans just grows and grows. Yet most people are completely unaware of their existence. Nor do they know what damage they are doing to body and psyche by living on a diet of convenience foods, which are empty of plant support. These health-enhancing compounds have come to be known as phytonutrients or neutraceuticals. They are perfect examples of what Hippocrates claimed more than 2,000 years ago – that certain foods are not only delicious but actually medicinal. And there are many: limonene which you find in citrus fruits, the isoflavone known as genistein in soy beans, allicin in onions and garlic.

Each has specific health-enhancing properties which are both powerful and deep acting. Some help lower

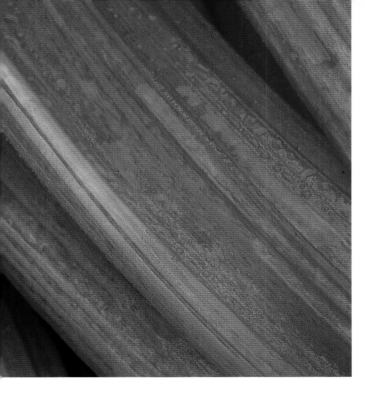

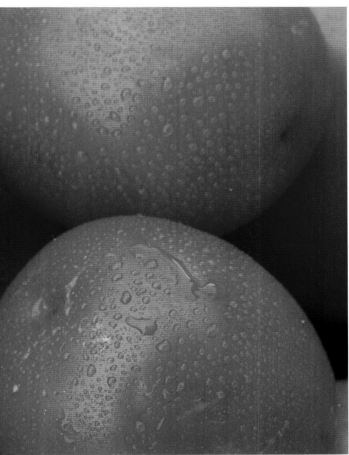

LDL cholesterol for instance. Some are strongly anti-cancer in their effects, or strengthen immunity. Others help clear the body of toxicity. Many, like the lignans in flax seeds, the flavonoids in the skins of oranges and grapefruits, and lycopene in tomatoes are superb antioxidants. As such, they are not only anti-agers protecting against free-radical damage, they even help rejuvenate the body in medically measurable ways and help guard against degenerative diseases like cancer, heart disease and diabetes. Scientists estimate that each of the 60 trillion cells in your body suffers 10,000 free-radical 'hits' each day. And this is on the up as a result of increasing chemicals in our environment. Phytonutrients help protect us from oxidation damage.

Surprising as it may seem, the antioxidant properties of many of these phytonutrients is greater than that of the vitamins A, C and E and the minerals selenium and zinc, which have become widely known as free radical scavengers. Use phytonutrients together with antioxidant vitamins and minerals and you get an unbeatable synergy. Make friends with the plant foods rich in phytonutrients. Try to build your daily meals around them. Eat as many of these foods as often as you can – raw, lightly steamed, or wok fried (see chart overleaf).

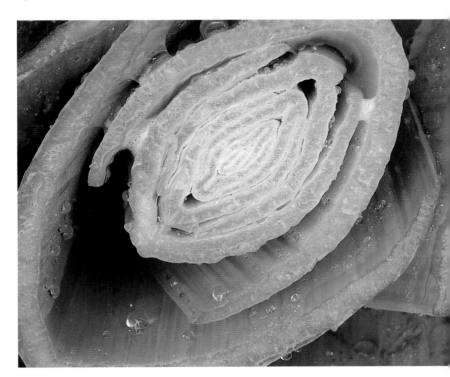

phytonutrient rich plants

plant	phytonutrients	benefits
garlic and onions	allyl sulfide (allicin)	◆ You will find potent antiviral and antibacterial properties in these vegetables. ◆ Allicin decreases the risk of stomach cancer and colon cancer, encourages the production of glutathione S-transferase – an enzyme that helps eliminate cancer-causing toxins from the body. ◆ These foods also offer many more useful anti-ageing and health promoting tasks.
green leafy vegetables: spinach, turnip, beet tops, collard greens, kale, also in yellow marrows or squashes	lutein	◆ A big league carotene antioxidant that resides in the fatty pigments of plants, lutein keeps carcinogens from binding to DNA and in doing so protects against degenerative diseases including eye diseases. ◆ It is the primary carotenoid present in the macula of the human retina. ◆ It also protects cells all over the body, including the skin, from premature ageing.
crucifers: broccoli, Brussels sprouts, cabbage, other leafy green vegetables	indoles sulforaphanes	◆ Indoles prevent cancer-causing hormones from attaching to cells by increasing your body's supply of the enzymes that weaken cancer-producing xeno-oestrogens. ◆ They also eliminate toxins and enhance immunity. ◆ Sulforaphanes remove carcinogens from cells and, in animal studies, even slow cancer growth.
soya products	isoflavones such as genistein, saponins and phytosterols. Caution: *Beware the aluminium content of soya.*	◆ Isoflavones – powerful antioxidants – protect against cancer, including breast cancer and early ageing. ◆ In addition, genistein is a plant oestrogen that helps protect from dangerous chemical oestrogens being taken up by the body's receptor sites. ◆ Japanese women who eat large quantities of soya-based products like tofu have only one-fifth the breast cancer incidence that American women do. ◆ Saponins enhance immune functions and bind to cholesterol, limiting its absorption in the intestines. ◆ Phytosterols in soya products lower elevated cholesterol.

plant	phytonutrients	benefits
tomatoes	lycopene P-coumaric acid coumarins	◆ A carotenoid, of the same famiy as beta-carotene, lycopene is one of the most potent antioxidants of all. ◆ Where it is high in the diet, colon and bladder cancer are low. ◆ the contents of tomatoes also help lower the risk of cardiovascular disease. ◆ P-coumaric acid (which you find in strawberries and peppers as well) inhibits the production of cancer-causing nitrosamines in the body. ◆ Coumarins reduce inflammation.
citrus fruits: oranges tangerenes grapefruits	lemonene glucarase	◆ Limonene increases your body's production of anti-cancer enzymes and enhances immunity. Glycarase deactivates cancer-causing degenerative chemicals that get into the body and eliminates them.
orange vegetables and fruits: mangos, pumpkins, carrots, sweet potatoes, squash marrows	alpha-carotene beta-carotene	◆ These vegetables get their colour from carotenes – antioxidants with a major capacity to boost general immunity and decrease the risk of many kinds of cancer as well as other degenerative diseases and premature ageing. (Other carotinoids in other foods such as lycopene, luetin, zeaxanthin and cryptoxanthin, may be equally important or even more valuable.)
berries, red grapes, red wine, artichokes, yams:	polyphenols	◆ Polyphenols lower the risk of heart disease and flush out cancer-causing chemicals. This group of phytochemicals includes the flavonoids that fight cell damage from oxidation, strengthen blood vessels, decrease the permeability of capillaries, protect the integrity of skin and improve the health of eyes.
Flax seed or linseed	lignan precursors	◆ Lignans are polyphenol antioxidants. Linseed (or flax seed) is chock full of lignan precursors – chemicals the body turns into lignans through its metabolic processes. They help prevent cancers including breast cancer by binding to oestrogen receptor sites, inhibiting oestrogen's cancer-producing activities. Flax seeds are also an excellent source of Omega-3 fatty acids important for the production of hormones.

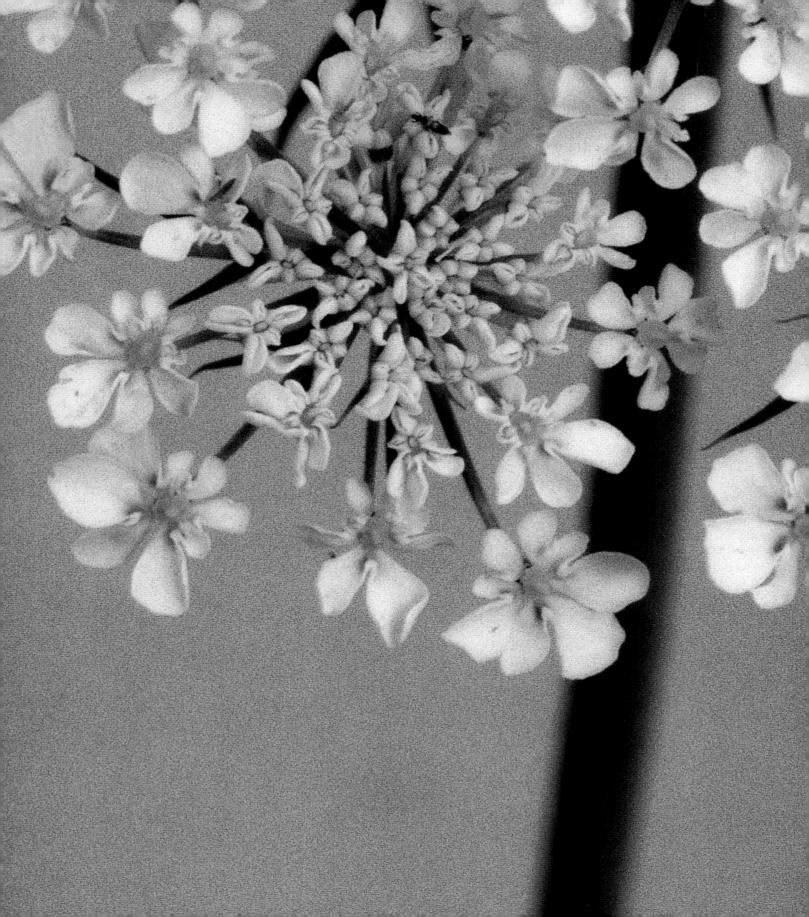

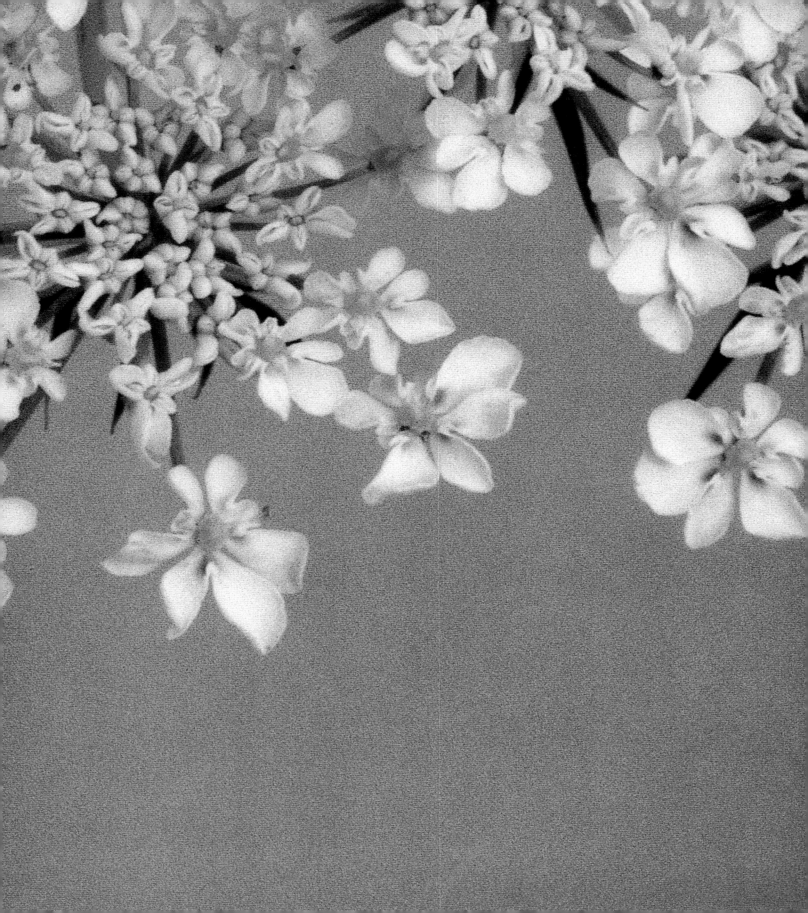

woman power

The balancing power of herbs brings

effective healing to women's ailments ...

From menstrual problems like PMS and endometriosis, to hot flushes and osteoporosis at menopause, herbs get to work. The herbs that balance the endocrine system (and so heal the female reproductive system) also enhance physical beauty thanks to their antioxidant and plant steroid contents.

Chinese angelica, black cohosh, dandelion, ginkgo, chasteberry, red clover, kava kava, yarrow, Queen Anne's Lace (wild carrot), marshmallow and ginger can help protect against premature ageing as well as degenerative diseases. Some, such as fenugreek, fennel and wild yam, can even be used to enlarge the breasts of women who are flat-chested. Get to know what they can do for you and you need never feel stuck in misery with nowhere to turn.

beware of oestrogens

Virtually every female problem is a manifestation of an underlying biochemical imbalance known as oestrogen dominance. It is really important to understand this. For oestrogen dominance is very much a product of the late twentieth century with all its environmental pollutants. Sadly, this is largely not understood by the medical profession, which is why so many doctors still prescribe oestrogen for female problems. While oestrogen given as a drug will indeed alleviate certain symptoms in many women – like hot flushes in menopause or amenorrhea in women of menstruating age – in reality taking it only masks the problem and in the long run it may lead to more serious problems, among them cancer of the breast and womb.

Oestrogen dominance is very much a symptom of our time. It has been brought about by the proliferation of petrochemically derived herbicides, pesticides and

◄ wild carrot

other chemicals in our environment, which are taken up by the body. There they behave as oestrogen-mimics in both men and women. Even the plastic cups we drink our tea and coffee from in the office, and the containers we use to cook foods in microwaves, leak chemical oestrogens so that we are constantly taking them into our bodies through our food and drink, even the air we breathe.

What this is doing to the male body is feminizing it. Environmentally absorbed chemical oestrogens are largely responsible for the huge drop in male sperm count in the West since the forties – almost 50% now of what it was then. In a female body, the results of being exposed to these powerful chemical oestrogens – and at the same time having even more prescribed for us by doctors in the form of the Pill and HRT – can be devastating. For the female reproductive system is some 20 times more complex than the male one.

get into balance

In a woman's body there are two major reproductive hormones: the oestrogens – of which there are three: E1, E2 and E3 – and progesterone. When oestrogen and progesterone are well balanced a woman does not suffer the common female problems – PMS, osteoporosis, fibroids, endometriosis or menopausal miseries – all of which have now become a widespread experience. Most of these ailments were rare in my mother's youth. Now they are becoming ubiquitous. When there is too much oestrogen and too little progesterone – which is the case in most women now – a woman's body becomes oestrogen dominant. Then, depending on her stage in life and whatever reproductive weaknesses she happens to have inherited from her ancestors, things start to go wrong. That is the bad news – very bad indeed as vast numbers of women are unaware of it and continue to fill their bodies with chemically based oestrogens – often at their doctor's insistence.

The good news is that herbs have much to offer as an alternative. Not only can they alleviate hard-to-treat problems like PMS and dry vagina in menopause, they also help get rid of the underlying cause by restoring the oestrogen-progesterone balance – indeed the entire highly complex hormonal symphony in a woman's body. Doing this in turn brings new energy, regeneration, rejuvenation and emotional balance. But be patient. It doesn't happen overnight. And you may have to experiment a bit with simple safe herbs to find out which help you most. There are so many to choose from. Most have been well tested and used for hundreds – sometimes thousands – of years.

trouble-free periods

In my experience the single most effective herb for regulating menstrual cycles is chastetree (*Vitex agnus-castus*). This plant gets its name because in the Middle Ages it was given to monks to banish lustful impulses – turning 'bad' monks into 'good' monks – thanks to its high content of oestrogenic plant steroids. But by no means does it cool the flames of desire in women.

Ancient Greek women gathered the pinwheel leaves of the chastetree, then plunged them into wine and gave it to their suffering sisters to regulate periods that were too short, too long or non-existent. In Europe, where we mostly use the berry from chastetree, it has long been the plant of choice for treating menstrual and menopausal difficulties. It has an ability to even out imbalances in reproductive hormones no matter what they may be and regardless of the time in a woman's life in which she experiences them.

The mechanisms of action of the chasteberry have been widely studied. One of the things it does is influence the pituitary gland to control the excess secretion of prolactin. Then irregular menstrual cycles tend to return to normal and PMS, menstrual cramps and other irregularities are alleviated.

Chastetree also helps with infertility. Like many of the hormone-balancing plants, this one is slow acting. So be patient. You may need to take it steadily for three months to reap its benefits fully. But once things are

rebalanced, you can often stop taking it altogether and remain symptom free – especially if your diet and health lifestyle are good.

Take agnus castus either as a tincture or a dried herb in capsules. Take ¼-½ teaspoon of tincture first thing in the morning in half a glass of water. But it is important that you not exceed this dose without being under the care of an experienced herbalist for chastetree is a very powerful plant. Chastetree works well with black cohosh, greater celandine and pasque flower for amenorrhea. In fact, it is sold this way in an excellent tincture in Germany called Femisana.

carrot cures

Known as wild carrot or Queen Anne's Lace (*Daucus carota*) happens to be one of the most beautiful meadow plants you will ever see. Not only are its seeds effective as an emmenagogue – a herb to bring on menstruation – the Pennsylvania Dutch have used wild carrot for two centuries to treat menstrual problems and as a morning-after contraceptive. Experiments with animals indicate that the plant does indeed have an ability to prevent implantation of a fertilized ova. This is probably thanks to a phytochemical it contains called phthalide, which helps trigger menstrual flow.

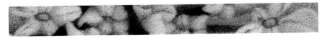

wild carrot tea

▶ *3 tsp dried wild carrot*
▶ *1 cup boiling water*

Pour the boiling water over the dried seeds and dried aerial parts of the wild carrot. Steep for 15 minutes. Strain and drink 1 cup three times a day. You can also take it in tincture form, ¼-½ teaspoon of the tincture three times a day in a glass of water.

Caution:
Chastetree is powerful enough to counteract the effects of the Pill in some women.

167

clear the spasms

One of the most uncomfortable problems associated with menstruation is cramps. They can show up either just before or during a period. A useful herb for getting rid of them is black haw (*Viburnum prunifolium*). Also known as cramp bark, this Native American remedy is related to the elder tree. It is both a sedative and an antispasmodic which acts as a muscle relaxant to the uterus when you take it.

Use this herb not on an on-going basis but only when you are experiencing period cramps to help relieve them. The bark of black haw boasts a number of phytochemicals to help soothe the womb and banish pain: aesculetin and scopoletin clear the spasm that causes the pain. The rest support the process in a synergistic manner by relaxing nervous tension.

black haw cream

▶ *1 tsp tincture of cramp bark*
▶ *50 g (2 oz) natural cream base (see Resources)*

Use this topically to help relieve pain. Mix the tincture with the natural cream base and apply to the belly and the back three or four times a day. Or take ½ teaspoon of tincture of cramp bark in ½ glass of water four to six times a day to relieve spasms.

chinese whispers

Another of my favourite herbs for just about every menstrual problem, including PMS, is Chinese angelica (*Angelica sinensis*), which is different to the European *Angelica archangelica*. The European variety has many of the same benefits but it tends to be a stimulant and does not have good antispasmodic abilities like its Chinese cousin. Also known as dang quai, Chinese angelica is one of the master herbs since it is also a tonic and an adaptogen as well.

Take up to ½ a teaspoon of dang quai tincture three times a day or make the root into wine. It is good for women of all ages on so many levels it would be hard to list them all. Like just about all of the hormonal balancing herbs, it combines well with others such as motherwort, passionflower and chastetree.

the spirit of motherwort

Its name betrays its nurturing nature. Motherwort (*Leonurus cardiaca*) brings a comforting sense of being gently cosseted in a loving mother's arms. It is an experience that makes you feel safe enough to allow deep change to take place without unnecessary anxiety or anguish. When it comes to improving your self-confidence and strengthening your ability to deal gracefully with life's ups and down, there is nothing quite like motherwort. It is a godsend when you feel your world has been pulled out from under you. Motherwort is a herb that reaches deep into the soul, touching the parts that other plants can't reach.

Motherwort can be a particularly valuable herb for women. It stimulates and promotes normal menstrual flow and is helpful to women who decide to come off the Pill. It can trigger delayed or suppressed menstruation – especially when stress, tension and anxiety are causing the problem. This is as much due to its ability to provide comfort as its ability to regulate hormones. It helps keep emotions on an even keel through all manner of hormonal upheaval, from menstruation to menopause.

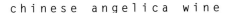

chinese angelica wine

► *100 g (4 oz) Chinese angelica root, chopped*
► *600 ml (1 pint) fruity white wine*

Place the chopped Chinese angelica root in a jar with a tight-fitting lid and cover it with the white wine (I like Muscatel best). Seal the mixture and put in a dark place for two weeks to steep, turning it over every day or two. At the end of this period, open the jar, strain off the herbs and rebottle the wine. Keep in a refrigerator for use. Take one wine-glass full a day on an empty stomach.

comfort and strength tea

► *2 tsp dried motherwort*
► *1 cup boiling water*

Collect the stalks of motherwort between early summer and autumn while its tiny flowers are in bloom and dry them thoroughly. They need to be gathered while the plant is flowering – June to September in the Northern Hemisphere, December to March in the Southern. Put the dried plant into a tea pot and pour the boiling water over it. Allow to steep for 15 minutes. Drink this tea three or four times a day during times of great change in your life and you will understand how this lovely plant with its three-part leaves got its common name. Alternatively, use 1 teaspoon of tincture in a little water three times a day.

Caution:
Avoid taking Chinese angelica while you are pregnant as it is a uterine stimulant. And while you are taking it be cautious about exposing yourself to excessive amounts of sunlight.

◄ chinese angelica

wings of desire

These days we treat aphrodisiacs as folk fantasy. Don't be deceived ...

They are very real indeed. The biochemistry of certain plants like ginseng, dang quai, fennel and wild yam, as well as certain essential oils can bring powerful sexual regeneration to the body and also intensify libido. It is your own individual response to specific herbs that is the key to aphrodisiacs. Loss of libido or impotence can have many different causes. So when turning to herbs for help in the sexual arena, you may need to experiment a bit to find which plants work best for you.

male potency

Sexual impotence or a loss of ability to maintain a full erection affects most men at some time in their life. It can be a result of feeling unwelcome, afraid of one's own power, or experiencing a sense of inadequacy or depression in life. Such things reflect themselves in the behaviour of your body. With real awareness of how each partner feels (even if he himself is still unaware of this) and with patience and consideration, psychologically caused impotence will often clear by itself. But many difficulties with maintaining erection are biochemical in nature. In men over the age of 35 it can happen during periods of prolonged stress, after illness, or simply as a result of having lived for too long on convenience foods. The body becomes depleted in essential minerals, trace elements and vitamins with the result that some of its metabolic processes no longer work properly.

The first step is to detoxify the body by doing a herbal cleanse. Then eliminate highly processed foods and eat lots of fresh vegetables and clean sources of protein (as outlined on pages 40-51). Also ensure you have a good supply of essential fatty acids, such as 2 to 3 tablespoons of flax seed oil each day, as they help produce the hormones needed for sexual potency.

power to the male

There are a number of plants you can use to enhance sexual energy and intensify erection.

Ginkgo biloba
This herb not only boosts the flow of blood to the brain but also to the penis, potentizing iffy erections. The best way to take it for this purpose is in the form of a very concentrated extract. Take between 50 and 250 mg a day. Do not take more since in large quantities gingko can cause loose bowels, nervousness and irritability. One research project gave men 80 mg of such a 50:1 extract three times a day and got good results. It not only cleared impotence, it also lifted the depression that often accompanies it. This is a very highly concentrated form of ginkgo and is not always readily available. You can instead use ginkgo tincture, 1 teaspoon in a little water three times a day.

Fava beans
Vicia faba can have an astounding effect on erection. The first written record of this food having sexual connotations came from ancient Rome, where Cicero used it to heighten his own passion. Fava is the best natural source of L-dopa. This chemical (which is also used to treat Parkinson's disease) intensifies erections in some men. That is how fava got its reputation as an aphrodisiac. One way to use fava is to sprout the beans for 8-10 days, washing them daily, and then eat the sprouts in salads or on their own.

Siberian ginseng
Eleutherococcus senticosus is a natural MAO inhibitor. It helps lift depression and improves libido in both men and women. It also helps overcome long-term fatigue. You can take it as an extract daily. Its effects build slowly over weeks and months. This adaptogen is an excellent restorative for the whole body.

woman in love

When libido flags in women there are all sorts of herbs that can help revive it.

Wild yam

Dioscorea villosa restores libido so successfully in most women that I would not advise you to use it unless you have a sexual partner. You can take the tincture – ½ -1 teaspoon in water three times a day – or as a dried herb in capsules, 4-6 capsules a day. I have known women to take 10 capsules a day, but less than this works very well for most. You can also make a cream or salve out of wild yam for vaginal dryness.

Add the extract (not the tincture, the alcohol would be irritating) to a cream base you have either bought or made (see page 144). Make your cream in a ratio of ¼ liquid extract to ¾ cream base – i.e. if you have 3 teaspoons of cream base, add 1 teaspoon of extract. A different way to do this is to buy a non-allergic vaginal lubricant, put it into a blender and whirr the extract into it. Comfrey cream is another excellent lubricant for vaginal dryness.

Chinese angelica

Angelica sinensis is the classic oriental treatment for low libido in women. Dang quai is a wonderful plant to use since it does so much good for your body and psyche all round while intensifying sexual desire. You can steep 3 to 6 teaspoons of the dried herb in 600 ml (1 pint) of boiling water for 20 minutes. Then strain and drink throughout the day.

Ginseng

Panax ginseng (various species) is as good a raiser of libido in women as it is in men despite the assumption that it is a male plant. It is particularly useful in post-menopausal women. Drink it as a tea three or four times a day.

Fennel

Foeniculum vulgare is replete with plant steroids. In animal experiments it raises the libido of both males and females. You can take it as a tea. Bruise 1 teaspoon of fennel seeds and pour 2 cups of boiling water over them. Steep for 5 minutes, strain and drink.

Other simple herbs that you can add to your foods that have a reputation for enhancing libido are parsley, fenugreek – great to sprout and eat in salads – ginger and anis (*Pimpinella anisum*). Even coca from which chocolate is made carries mild aphrodisiac power.

Essential oils

These help with libido on the night. Massage your body and that of your partner with an oil to which you have added one of the aphrodisiac essences: try clary sage, ylang ylang, rose, or jasmine. This is for external use only. They are powerful stuff. You need only 1 drop of essential oil to each teaspoon of a pure vegetable oil such as sweet almond oil or apricot oil. A capsule of vitamin E squeezed into the oil when you mix it helps keep it fresh longer.

Cautions:

Chinese angelica is not a herb to use when you are pregnant

Do not use fennel oil on your body when you are pregnant as it can cause miscarriage.

the great passage

It is a time when you are able to let go of the roles that have defined your life – wife, lover, mother, whatever – and move deep into your own being to discover who you really are at a soul level and what your life is about from here on out. Yet, for many women the passage to creativity, energy and freedom is not an easy one. Oestrogen-mimicking hormones in the environment – known as xenoestrogens – may have made her body oestrogen dominant with all the miseries this can imply. She may be tired after half a life of hard work or struggle. She may feel lost or confused about who she is and where she is going. She may be worried about hot flushes or sleepless nights, changes in her body or in her feelings.

The passage of menopause demands that you go deep, deep within on both a physical and a spiritual level. It asks that you move towards a way of living which is more authentic to the nature of your being. There are literally dozens of plants that can accompany you during this profound period of change – plants that offer side-effect-free hormone replacement, plants to rejuvenate your body, plants to cleanse and plants to rebalance hormones and eliminate symptoms such as night sweats or dry vagina. There are even plants that seem willing to hold your hand like a best friend for safety and comfort while you make this life-changing journey.

natural HRT is best

Oestrogen drugs given in HRT immediately relieve certain symptoms associated with menopause such as hot flashes and vaginal dryness. But using them is rather like continuing to take aspirin for a headache day after day instead of dealing with its cause so you don't need aspirin any more. Oestrogen drugs increase your risk of breast cancer and carry other potentially harmful side-effects. Finally, when you take HRT – for hot flushes for instance – you have to continue taking it. For the moment you get off of it, whether that be a few months or many years down the road, the hot flushes come back with full force.

Herbs are slower to clear problems but they go far deeper. They don't just mask symptoms. I believe the only reason doctors don't encourage a natural approach to menopausal help is that most of them simply do not know it is possible. Pharmaceutical companies are interested not in providing information about natural menopause but rather in making a profit on the drugs they sell. Much of the money they spend on product promotions is spent 'educating' doctors about the value of their drugs. And sadly that is all the 'education' most busy doctors get.

phyto-promises

Hot flushes and night sweats erupt as a result of the rapid decrease in oestrogen in a woman's body around the time of menopause. This is the reason for vaginal dryness too. Yet such symptoms are practically non-existent in Asian cultures – that is until Western convenience foods become widespread. People living largely on natural plants such as fresh vegetables and fruits and beans – especially soya beans – very rarely experience them. Beans and some other plants contain phytochemicals which have mild oestrogenic effects: lignans, phytosterols, saponins and isoflavones for instance.

These plant chemicals are very mild in their actions. They are nothing like the dangerous petrochemically derived xenoestrogens in our environment nor the oestrogen drugs used in HRT. Yet they have an effective hormonal balancing and protective effect on the body. They are taken up by oestrogen receptor sites, into which they fit like a key in a lock. There they not only modulate any loss of oestrogen as a result of the loss of production of this hormone by the ovaries, they also block much of the uptake of the dangerous xenoestrogens. They help guard the body from oestrogen dominance and the Pandora's box of conditions – from cancer of the womb to osteoporosis – that can result from it. Plants have the unique ability to balance the body.

That is how these plant chemicals can help lower the burden of oestrogen dominance in a woman who is carrying it while in someone who needs extra oestrogen they can supply it in a safe and simple to use form. Not only when you are approaching menopause but all though your life try to put a few organic – not genetically modified – soya-based products in your life by eating some organic tofu, using organic tamari or soy sauce as seasoning and using organic soya milk as a base for soups and drinks. One of my favourite ways to introduce phytoestrogens into a woman's life is to suggest that she combines phyto-steroid-rich foods to make a delicious and quick breakfast.

plant hormones

There are many herbs with this balancing ability too. Either on their own or in combination they create a truly natural method for HRT – slowly but inexorably clearing unpleasant symptoms, strengthening the organism as a whole, and making your passage a more graceful one. These same plants also help balance emotions. So

perfect quick breakfast or meal replacement

▶ ⅓ cup blanched almonds
▶ ⅔ cup soya milk
▶ 1 ripe banana
▶ few drops vanilla essence
▶ 2 tsp honey

Blend the almonds and soya milk really well until the mixture is smooth. Then add the other ingredients and process well. Serve immediately.

important are they that I would advise every woman – no matter what her age – to learn about them, use them, grow those that can be grown in her home climate, and make friends with them all.

natural replacement

There are so many plants that offer natural hormone replacement that a woman is almost spoiled for choice in deciding which ones to use. And, provided you are patient, in my experience they will sort out your miseries effectively and in a life-empowering way. Many of these same plants bring relief from what I call menopausal syndrome, which includes all sorts of symptoms you are better off without: hot flushes, night sweats, depression, anxiety, vaginal dryness, palpitations, forgetfulness and irregular menstruation.

In Chinese medicine this syndrome is associated with a deficiency of kidney qi – basic life energy. A chemical-free natural diet rich in fresh vegetables, phyto-steroids and antioxidant plant factors plus good low-fat protein and herb support will gently but deeply transform the way you look and feel, clearing symptoms and creating a new vision of yourself, your life and your future. Plants such as wild yam, passionflower, lady's slipper, fennel, fenugreek, celery stalks, elder, liquorice, false unicorn root, dates, alfalfa, chastetree and red clover are all rich in phyto-oestrogens. As well as offering natural hormone balance and support when you need it most, they supply vitality. You can use them individually. Often they work even better in combination.

luscious liquorice

Like soya, liquorice (*Glycyrrhiza glabra*) is replete with natural oestrogenic plant chemicals, especially glycyrrhizin, the plant's most active ingredient. It is deliciously sweet – 50 times sweeter than sugar. Glycyrrhizin helps to lower oestrogen in women when it is too high and to increase the 'right' kind of oestrogen when the body needs more. But before you run out to buy more liquorice sweets, they won't do it. You need to use the roots of this herb in the form of a decoction: three cups a day, or as a tincture: ½ teaspoon twice a day in a little water. Liquorice has a bonus in that, when it

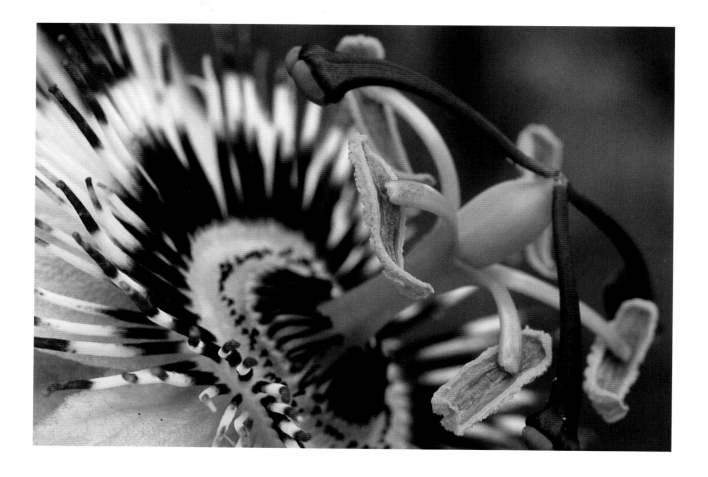

comes to rebuilding your energy, it offers powerful adrenal support – valuable to any woman under long-term stress – and enhances the functioning of the immune system.

Caution:
Do not use liquorice if you have high blood pressure nor during pregnancy.

pause for tea

You can make a light, good-tasting tea of alfalfa leaves and drink it several times a day. Red clover makes another pleasant-tasting tea for natural HRT. It contains between 1 and 3% isoflavones – gentle, neutral, plant oestrogens. In a study where menopausal women were given a combination of flax seed, clover and soya – even for as short a period as two weeks – the levels of oestrogen in their bodies increased significantly. It is the

alfalfa tea

▶ *4 tsp fresh alfalfa or 2 tsp dried*
▶ *1 cup boiling water*

Steep the herb in a cup of boiling water for 10 minutes. Strain and drink.

he shou wu tea

▶ *50 g (2 oz) he shou wu*
▶ *900 ml (1½ pints) water*

Make a decoction of he shou wu by steeping the herb in the water and drink glasses of it throughout the day. Alternatively, turn it into a medicinal wine (see page 35).

oestrogenic nature of clover that gives farmers trouble, by the way. If cows eat too much of some varieties the animals can spontaneously abort a pregnancy.

use a tonic

False unicorn root is a good overall glandular tonic. It stimulates ovarian hormones and is helpful both in early menopause and especially after hysterectomy. There is also a useful Chinese plant called he shou wu (*Polygonum multiflorum*), which you can buy in any shop that sells oriental herbs. It is a great blood tonic – particularly useful in early menopause. It also counteracts the tendency many women of menopausal age have towards constipation.

oestrogens from nature

Two of my favourite plant hormone herbs are fenugreek (*Trigonella foenum-graecum*) and wild yam (*Dioscorea villosa*). Both contain a lot of a particular phytochemical called diosgenin, which was originally used by drug companies to convert into synthetic progestogen drugs. Fenugreek has more of this phytochemical than does wild yam. It is also a great detoxifier. Whatever else you

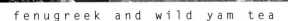

fenugreek and wild yam tea

▶ *50 g (2 oz) fenugreek seeds*
▶ *50 g (2 oz) wild yam root*
▶ *900 ml (1½ pints) boiling water*
▶ *pinch basil, liquorice, cumin (opitonal)*
▶ *1 lemon*
▶ *honey*

Steep the fenugreek seeds and wild yam root in the boiling water for 20 minutes. Then add a pinch of basil, liquorice and cumin if you have it and squeeze the juice of a lemon and add honey to taste. Chill and drink three wine glasses of it a day.

◀ passionflower

do, drink fenugreek regularly as a tea. It's delicious. Wild yam is a wonderfully strengthening plant to the whole system while it offers excellent hormone balancing. What may surprise you is that for centuries these herbs have also been used successfully by women with small breasts to enlarge them. It really does work for many, especially when you combine these two herbs with other natural oestrogenic plants like fennel, cumin and liquorice. My own recipe for this is given opposite.

get into black

The most well-documented natural alternative to hormone replacement therapy is black cohosh (*Cimicifuga racemosa*). Recent research shows that it performs at least as well as drugs. In one eight-week study of 110 menopausal women, half took black cohosh root extract while the others were given a placebo. Afterwards, blood tests showed significant oestrogenic activity. In another study comparing women taking this herb with others on drug-based HRT, scientists found that the relief from symptoms such as hot flushes and vaginal dryness was equal in both groups.

Black cohosh lowers luteinizing hormone (LH). An increase in LH production is a major underlying reason for many menopausal miseries. This wonderful plant is effective for hot flushes, night sweats, depression, anxiety, lowered libido and vaginal atrophy. No wonder it is the best-selling herbal product in Germany.

It works well to mix tincture of motherwort – which supports deep spiritual and psychological change – together with tincture of black cohosh. Use one part black cohosh to 2 parts motherwort. Take ¼ to ½ teaspoon in half a glass of water three times a day. Very occasionally black cohosh can cause a tummy upset. If this happens, decrease the amount or replace it with one of the other menopausal-helper herbs.

plant-based HRT

Over the years I have experimented on myself and with others using many individual herbs as well as mixtures. Both can alleviate menopausal symptoms and act as natural HRT, balancing hormones in a woman's body. However, each woman is unique in her biochemistry. It

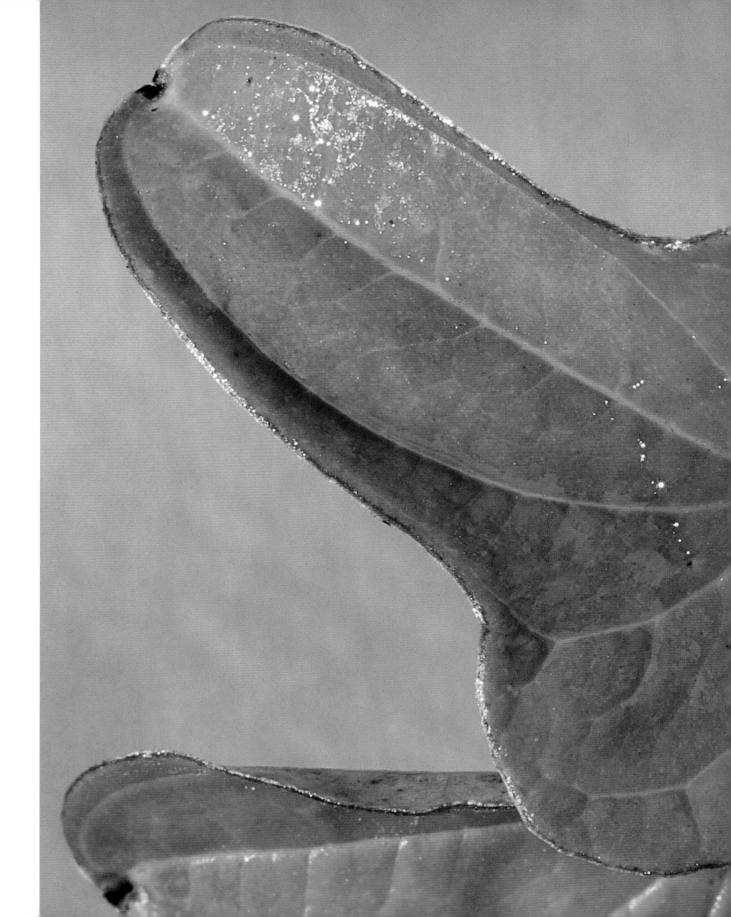

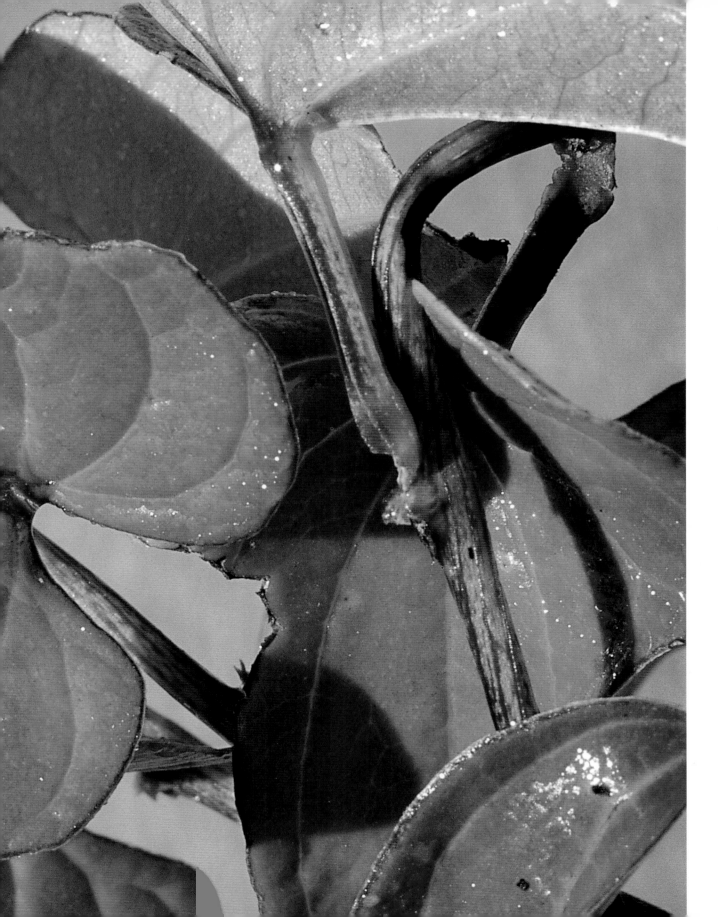

can take some trial and error to find out which plants work best for you. This means taking a particular plant or plant combination for a period of six weeks to three months, although many women experience benefits far sooner and a few immediately.

Once you find the right herb and have continued to take it for from three to eighteen months, it is likely that you will not need it any more. It will have performed its balancing act and your body can take over itself from there. I like using blends of different herbs to help women handle menopause. In that way you can get the synergistic effect where the whole of the blend is greater than any of its parts. It also seems to me (although I have no scientific explanation or even confirmation for this) that, when supplied with a variety of plants – all of which have hormonal balancing properties – a woman's body quite naturally makes first use of those that she needs most. This often brings about faster results and, in the case of some women, goes far deeper in its actions. Here are my favourite three formulas for menopausal symptoms and natural HRT.

The first is a tincture mix made from herbal tinctures you buy ready-made. It is especially helpful at the onset of menopausal symptoms. Use it together with a diet that cuts out convenience foods and anything else containing sugar or processed fats. Be sure to get plenty of good protein either from vegetarian sources or by taking eggs, organic meat, free-range chicken and fresh fish. And beware of dairy products including milk and yoghurt and cheese (butter is alright taken in moderate

leslie's menopause mix

▶ *1 part tincture of liquorice*
▶ *1 part tincture of dandelion root*
▶ *1 part tincture of wild yam*
▶ *2 parts tincture of motherwort*
▶ *1 part tincture of sage*

Mix together the tinctures and funnel into a clean bottle. Shake well before use each time. Take ½ teaspoon in half a glass of water four times a day. When symptoms clear gradually decrease the amount until you stop altogether.

◀ wild yam

leslie's HRT tincture

▶ *25 g (1 oz) wild yam root*
▶ *25 g (1 oz) black cohosh*
▶ *25 g (1 oz) dandelion root*
▶ *25 g (1 oz) liquorice root*
▶ *25 g (1 oz) Chinese angelica (dang quai)*
▶ *50 g (2 oz) fenugreek seeds*
▶ *3 cups alcohol*
▶ *1 cup distilled or spring water*

Put the herbs into a big jar with a top that will seal and pour the alcohol and distilled or spring water over them. Cover the mixture and store in a cool place for two weeks making sure to shake the jar a couple of times each day. Then put the mixture in a cafetière and press firmly to extract as much of the herbal goodness a possible. Finally filter through muslin or a jelly bag and pour the strained liquid into a clean jar or bottle for storage. (The herbal residue that you throw away makes great compost for the garden by the way.) I store my tinctures in the refrigerator. It is partly my childhood spent in the United States where we refrigerate just about everything and partly because I like tinctures cold rather than at room temperature. Take 1 teaspoon of this mixture three to four times each day.

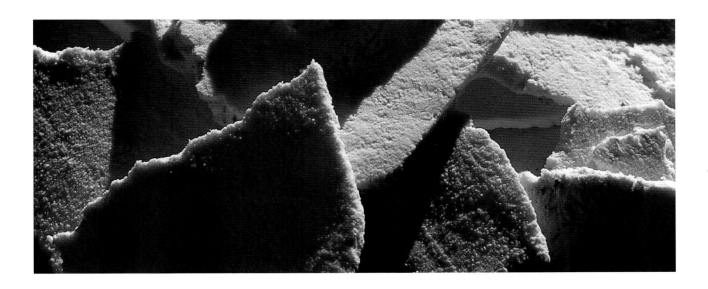

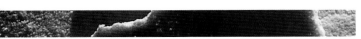

leslie's woman's tea

▶ *50 g (2 oz) horsetail*
▶ *75 g (3 oz) chasteberry*
▶ *75 g (3 oz) red clover*
▶ *75 g (3 oz) motherwort*
▶ *75 g (3 oz) Chinese angelica (dang quai)*
▶ *25 g (1 oz) Siberian ginseng*
▶ *900 ml (1½ pints) boiling water*
▶ *finely grated rind of 1 organic orange or lemon or 2 organic tangerines*

Mix the herbs together well, being sure to crush any in large pieces. You can use a mortar and pestle for this if you like, or put them in a coffee grinder. Infuse 25 g (1 oz) of the blend in the boiling water, cover and steep for 30 minutes. Strain and refrigerate. Drink a glass full of this mixture three times a day.

quantities) and of wheat. Many women's bodies don't handle them well.

The second is a home-made tincture specifically formulated as a natural HRT product. It uses herbs that revive the adrenals, provide a good supply of plant-based steroids with oestrogenic activity and strengthen both mind and body. Make it yourself by steeping the dried herbs in a mixture of 75% alcohol and 25% water. It will keep for up to two years. It is very inexpensive as you can buy these herbs in small quantities. (I keep any leftover dried herbs in a moisture-free, sealed container in the refrigerator or even in the freezer to preserve their active properties for as long as possible.) You can use vodka to make it if you like although I prefer rum, since I find it masks the unpleasant taste of certain plants. Use dried herbs and make sure that the root herbs are in small pieces before you make your mixture so their ingredients are more readily absorbed into the alcohol and water.

If you prefer a tea, the third recipe is the best I have ever found. In addition to oestrogenic plants it contains horsetail, which is high in silicon, to help strengthen your bones, nails, skin and hair; motherwort for courage and comfort during deep life transitions; and orange and lemon rind for flavour. Make it from top quality dried herbs. Take the herbs and mix them together in a jar.

▲ wild yam extract

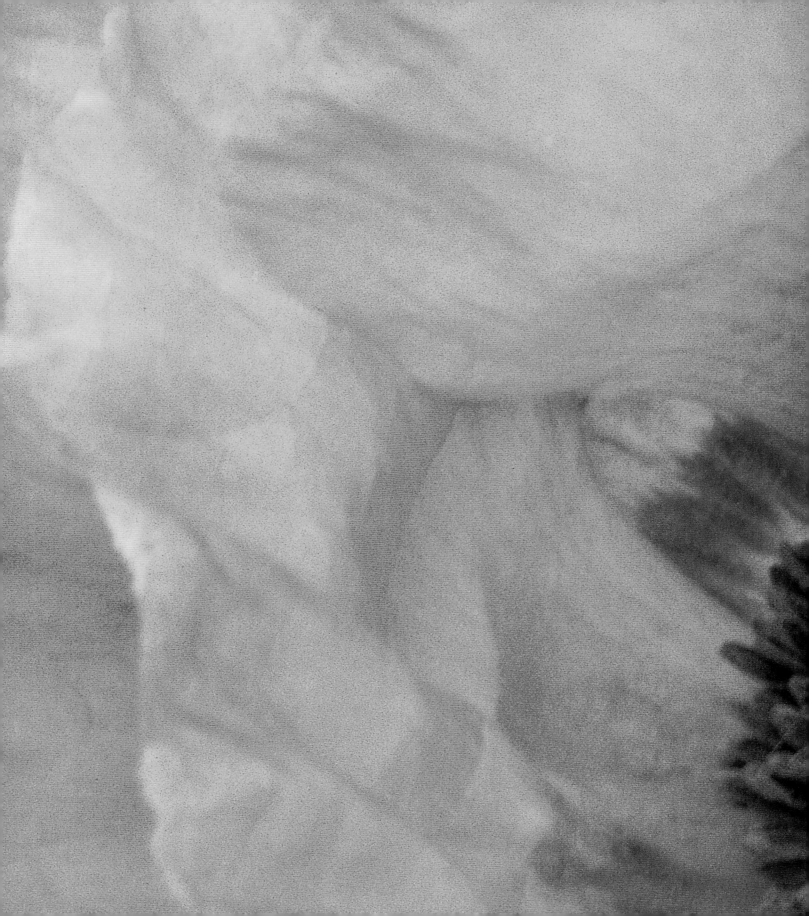

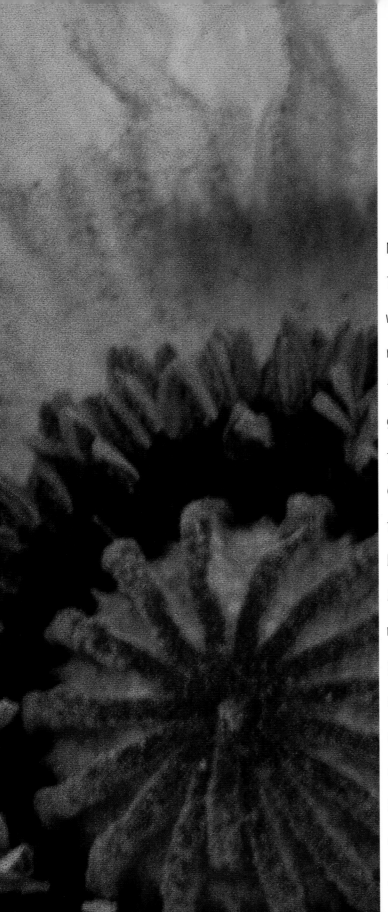

banishing

⁸

banishing

Nowhere do plants offer more love and care than in their willingness to help when you need fast relief. And they do it with such ease. Here is my guide to the simplest remedies for banishing everything from colds to hangovers, headaches to head lice. It includes a basic first aid kit (see page 207) to help you deal with minor emergencies and niggling problems. For in banishing aches and pains, irritations and injuries, the sacred power of herbs expresses itself with breathtaking simplicity, efficiency and depth.

◄ poppy

aches and pains

Pain is what many people fear the most. We all know the misery that can come from a sore back, a throbbing headache or toothache, not to mention children's earaches. All too many also know the immobilizing pain of migraine. Herbs can reach out and help when pain strikes, and without the upset stomach and muzzy heads that over-the-counter treatments can bring in their wake.

symptom	what to use	how to use it
Backache We've all done it – picked up something too heavy or twisted awkwardly – and suffered the pain of an indignant back. Essential oils really come into their own with back pain, use them to relieve muscle spasm and ease your mind.	◆ Essential oils of sage, thyme and rosemary all contain thymol and carvacrol, which are excellent muscle relaxants. Rosemary has the added advantage of being antispasmodic. Clary sage is also used traditionally to ease the pain of a pulled back.	◆ You can mix a few drops of one of these essential oils with a couple of tablespoons of almond oil. Either massage it into the sore spot yourself or allow someone you trust to do it gently for you. A warm bath will also help ease the tightness out of strained back muscles. Put a few drops of essential oil of rosemary or clary sage in the bath plus 2 cups of industrial grade Epsom salts (available from your chemist). Allow the essential oils to vaporize on the steam to help you relax all over. Stay in the bath for half an hour, topping up with hot water, to let the Epsom salts do their muscle-relaxing work (see also page 63).
Earache Earache is just as bad as toothache in that you can never seem to get at the pain.	◆ Warm garlic infused oil is something you can make yourself (see page 75) and keep to hand. It is soothing and will help see off any infection in your ear. 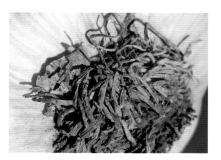	◆ Put a small amount of garlic infused oil – never essential oil of garlic, it would be far too strong – in a spoon and warm it over a gas ring or candle until it is comfortably warm and not hot. Suck it into an ear dropper and put two drops into the ear. Plug with cotton wool and repeat every hour until the pain has gone. Caution: *Don't use this remedy for swimmer's ear as it will increase the irritation, and don't use it ever if you think you have a punctured ear drum or an external ear infection.*

symptom	what to use	how to use it

Hangover

The most obvious way to avoid a hangover is don't drink. If you do drink then choose only the best – be it wine, whisky, vodka, whatever. The best always has fewer unpleasant chemicals to upset the system. Drinking lots of fluids along with the alcohol also helps to prevent the dehydration that comes with an over-indulgent evening. If you get it wrong, however, there are a few things you can do in the morning to make you feel better.

◆ First thing in the morning after make yourself a cup of peppermint tea (see page 57).

◆ The peppermint will settle your stomach. Breathing in the steam from your tea will help to ease your headache. If it persists then take a look at the headache remedies overleaf.

◆ When your stomach is settled enough to handle more, take a couple of grams of vitamin C and 2-3 grams of evening primrose oil or star flower. The vitamin C's antioxidant properties help the liver clear the toxic wastes from too much alcohol. The GLA in these oils is turned into prostaglandin E1. This is a very important regulator of mood in the body which alcohol depletes. When it is low you tend to feel depressed and very tired.

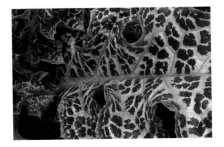

◆ Milk thistle is also a wonderful liver cleanser (see page 66-9).

◆ Take 2 capsules or 1 teaspoon of tincture in a little water every 3-4 hours until you are feeling better.

◆ If you can remember where you last saw it in your current state, reach for some dried borage as well.

◆ Open the jar, or put it in a paper bag, hold your nose over the bag and take a deep breath. No one has ever explained to me how it does it, but it clears your head wonderfully.

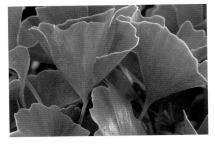

◆ I have heard that taking ginkgo before you go out also helps to prevent hangovers by enhancing your body's ability to metabolize alcohol swiftly. However, I've never heard anyone say how much you should take, or how long before drinking alcohol you should take it. If you are taking ginkgo for other reasons, pay attention to how you feel after a glass or two of wine and see if it makes a difference.

symptom	what to use	how to use it

Headaches

Headaches can be caused by anything from eating something that disagrees with you to nervous tension. If you have frequent headaches, find yourself a good herbalist to get to the root of the problem. If you only get a headache from time to time, here are a few fast and furious remedies to cut through the pain and let you get on with your day.

◆ Willow bark (*Salix alba*) contains a phytochemical called salicin. This breaks down in the body to produce salicylic acid – the chemical supplied by aspirin. What willow bark appears to do is to block the production of certain prostaglandins in the body which cause pain and inflammation. It is an excellent form of pain relief. Commission E, who advise the German Government about herbs, are 100% behind the use of willow bark for pain relief. Never take willow bark with aspirin or alcohol, and check with your doctor before using it if you are taking any other medication. Do not give it to children, it carries the same dangers as aspirin.

◆ Put 1 teaspoon of powdered or crushed bark into a tea pot and pour a cup of boiling water over it. Let it steep for 15-20 minutes and drink. Mixing a little caffeine with aspirin increases the aspirin's effectiveness, possibly because of caffeine's ability to constrict blood vessels. You might like to try following your willow bark tea with a cup of green tea for added pain relief.

Caution: *Like aspirin, willow bark irritates the stomach in some people (although unlike aspirin, it passes through the stomach before turning into salicylic acid). If this is the case, drink it only with meals or use another form of pain relief.*

◆ I keep a little bottle of essential oil of peppermint near me wherever I go. Peppermint oil contains a widely recognized pain reliever, menthol. It acts by first stimulating then suppressing the nerves that feel pain.

◆ Rub a tiny amount on your forehead or temples whenever you feel a headache coming on. Be careful not to get it anywhere near your eyes as it burns. And wash your hands immediately to avoid touching sensitive parts of your body.

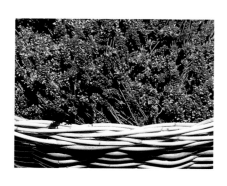

◆ When I have a busy schedule when I am travelling I make up a little bottle of my Headache Banisher to sniff gently at the first sign of a headache. I find that even the action of stopping to breathe deeply helps ward off a tension headache. Meanwhile the essential oils clear my head, allowing me to think more clearly.

◆ Into a small bottle put 10 drops of essential oil of lavender, 10 drops oil of essential oil of peppermint, 5 drops of essential oil of cloves. Sniff whenever you need it.

◆ Another lovely head freshener is rose vinegar. I make a little of this each summer from my favourite roses in the garden. I put a few drops on to my handkerchief if I have a headache, or rub a little into my temples.

◆ Put 300 ml (½ pint) cider vinegar into a small jar and toss in 25 g (1 oz) in weight of your favourite rose petals. Leave the jar in the airing cupboard for 10 days. Then strain the vinegar and bottle it.

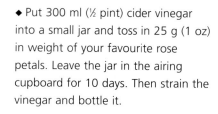

symptom	what to use	how to use it

Headaches cont.

◆ If you suffer from tension headaches consider learning a relaxation technique or two, joining a yoga class, or having a regular massage. In the short term, just stop and concentrate on making a cup of herb tea. This ritual alone can help to ease the tension before the tea ever reaches your lips. Calming teas like camomile or passionflower will ease the emotional tension, lavender will help with physical symptoms

◆ To make lavender tea, put 2 teaspoons of fresh lavender flowers or a teaspoon of the dried herb into a tea pot. Pour over a cup of boiling water, steep for 10 minutes, strain and drink.
◆ You can also put a drop of essential oil of lavender behind each ear, at the back of the head at the base of the spine on either side, and on each temple (keep your hands and the oil well away from your eyes). Or put 3 or 4 drops of lavender essential oil into your bath, lie back, and relax that headache away.

Migraine

To most of the one-in-ten people in the West who suffer from migraine, the only alternative to excruciating pain is the side-effects of anti-migraine drugs. Herbs – especially feverfew – provide a safe alternative.

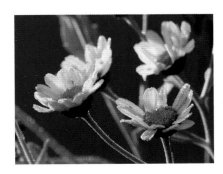

◆ Feverfew is a bright, irrepressible little plant that packs a big anti-migraine punch. Studies show that it inhibits the effects of migraine-related chemicals produced by the body, including histamines. Feverfew's vasodilatory effects also help ease the constricted blood flow associated with migraines. Meanwhile, its relaxing properties help you let go during an attack. Feverfew works best as a preventative measure.

◆ Try taking a couple of feverfew capsules each day. Chewing the fresh leaves is another way to reap the plant's prophylactic properties. Feverfew's leaves have anti-inflammatory and antispasmodic properties. They don't just relieve the symptoms; they actually inhibit the prostaglandins that are responsible for inflammation and pain. But eating the plant's leaves can cause mouth ulcers. My friends who do this place two or three leaves between two slices of bread to make a sandwich (use 100% rye bread if you suspect you are sensitive to wheat) to prevent irritation to the mouth.

◆ If migraine strikes, try taking tincture of willow bark rather than your usual over-the-counter pain killer.

◆ The tincture has a stronger effect than drinking willow bark tea, and is much easier to use than having to juggle with boiling water and tea pots when your vision is disturbed. Take 1 teaspoon of willow bark tincture in water every 2 hours until the pain goes.

symptom	what to use	how to use it
Migraine cont.	◆ At the onset of a migraine, blood vessels to the brain become constricted, bringing on the visual disturbances, confusion and pain characteristic of migraine. Taken regularly, rosemary, ginkgo and ginger can each work against this constriction and help bring relief from some of the symptoms migraine sufferers dread. See which one works for you.	◆ **Rosemary:** drinking rosemary tea daily helps to keep blood vessels dilated. To make rosemary tea put 1 teaspoon of the dried herb in a tea pot and pour a cup of boiling water over it. Steep for 10 minutes, strain and drink. ◆ **Ginkgo:** *Ginkgo biloba* improves blood supply to the brain by strengthening blood vessels. It also helps to prevent the blood vessels constricting. Take 1 capsule three times a day as a preventative measure. ◆ **Ginger:** drinking ginger tea daily keeps blood flowing smoothly by stopping blood vessels from dilating. Make ginger tea by grating 12 mm (½ in) of the root into a tea pot and pouring a cup of boiling water over it. Steep for 5-10 minutes, strain and drink.
	◆ Allowing yourself to relax during a migraine can help to relieve some of the pain, but relaxing is often the last thing you can do. Resting your head on a herb pillow can be pleasantly soothing and may help you get some sleep.	◆ Make a herb sachet (see page 94) and stuff it with equal quantities of dried lavender, marjoram, hops and peppermint leaves. Use it when you most need its help.
Toothache The only way to cure toothache is to see your dentist. Until you can get there, however, there are certain herbs you can call upon to stop the pain driving you up the wall.	◆ Try using essential oil of cloves	◆ Rubbed on to the aching tooth this will anaesthetize the whole area. Cloves contain eugenol, which deadens pain. Don't over-use it or you can burn the gum.
	◆ Alternatively, look to sesame seeds; they are loaded with pain-relieving phytochemicals.	◆ To get at the phytochemicals, make a strong tea by boiling 4 teaspoons of sesame seeds in a cup of water for a few minutes. Cool and pour into a jar without straining. Soak one end of a cotton-bud with the liquid and apply to the tooth and surrounding gum.

colds and flu

The common cold, believe it or not, can be associated with any one of up to 200 different viruses. No wonder it's so easy to end up with one. The best way to deal with colds and flu is not to get them in the first place: see Antiviral Power (pages 74-83).

symptom	what to use	how to use it

Soothing treatments

If, despite your best efforts, you wake up one morning with the characteristic scratchy throat and heavy-back-of-the-nose feeling, act fast. There are many antiviral herbs, not to mention herbs that soothe and comfort, that quickly beat colds or flu into submission if you use them straight away.

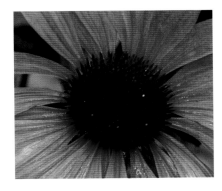

◆ At the first sign of a cold, reach for tincture of echinacea. It acts quickly (more quickly than taking capsules) to kill bacteria and boost your immune system. Western medicine has searched for a cure for the common cold like the knights of the round table searched for the grail. Here is one possibility, a plant with a two-pronged effect – to directly fight bacterial and viral infections while boosting the immune system at the same time.

◆ Take a teaspoon in water every hour or two for the first day. Then take 1 or 2 teaspoons three or four times a day until the symptoms are gone (see also pages 78-9).

◆ Follow this with some elderberry tincture. For the flu virus to really get a hold it has to reproduce in your body. This it can only do within the cells. A flu virus has spikes on its surface which it uses to puncture cells and break into them. It appears that elderberry knocks the spikes off, so it is unable to reproduce and can't get a firm hold on your system.

◆ Take ½-1 teaspoon in water every 4 hours. Continue to take elderberry at 4-hourly intervals for the next three days to make sure all of the virus has been immobilized (see also page 83)

◆ Get into C.

◆ Take 2 g of vitamin C straight away. Repeat this dose three times a day so you are taking 6 g a day until your cold has cleared. The body flushes out whatever vitamin C it doesn't need so if you find your stools are loose, cut back the dose. You will find when your body is fighting off a cold or flu it is likely to use all the vitamin C it can get.

symptom	what to use	how to use it

Soothing treatments cont.

◆ Have a cup of herb tea to get your circulation going. If your blood is moving smoothly around your body, it will be able to pass the infection from your system that much quicker. Make your tea from something you have to hand, don't wait until you get a chance to shop. Choose from: yarrow, peppermint, elderflower, camomile, lemon balm, lemon verbena, sage, thyme, rosemary, or basil.

◆ Steep 1 teaspoon of the dried herb in a cup of boiling water for 5-10 minutes. Use 2 teaspoons of the fresh leaves or flowers if you have them. Add a good dollop of honey to your tea – it kills bacteria.

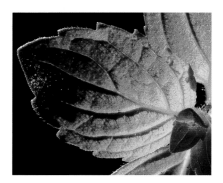

◆ If you can't sleep, try camomile and peppermint tea – they clear your head and relax you. These herbs are especially effective in a steam inhalation.

◆ 1 teaspoon of each dried herb to 1 cup of boiling water, steep for 5 minutes, strain and drink.
◆ Alternatively, put your herbs in a bowl rather than a tea pot and pour boiling water over them. Lean over the pan and put a towel over your head to make a 'tent' over the bowl. Breath in the vapours while your tea steeps. Then strain your tea and drink.

◆ Make yourself some chicken soup – yes really. It appears our grandmothers were absolutely right. Use vegetable stock or Marigold Swiss Vegetable Bouillon Powder (see Resources) if you are vegetarian.

◆ Make your soup with lots of fresh vegetables. Go heavy on the onion, which is good for colds. Add a generous pinch of thyme and sage. They go well with chicken and they are also antimicrobial and antiseptic. Just before serving, crush as much garlic as you can stand and add it to the pot to clear your head and boost your immune system. Garnish liberally with watercress. It too helps dry a runny nose.
◆ If you feel too ill to make soup, cook a whole, peeled onion in just enough soya milk or rice milk to cover. Simmer at a low heat until it is tender. Then drink the hot milk and eat the onion – delicious!

Soothing treatments cont.

◆ Put your feet in a hot mustard bath. I always thought this was a joke until I tried it. It is relaxing, warming and a real treat.

◆ Put 1 tablespoon of ordinary mustard powder into a foot bath or large pan. Slowly fill it with hot water, stirring well (don't pour it all at once or the mustard will go into lumps). Put your feet into the bath and soak for 20 minutes. Top up with more hot water whenever the water starts to cool.

◆ A hot bath with essential oils is also tremendously soothing.

◆ Take a long, hot bath and add 3 or 4 drops of tea tree oil or manuka oil to the water. They both have helpful antiseptic properties. While you wallow in the tub sip a cup of willow bark tea (see page 208) to ease a throbbing head and soothe the aches that come with flu.

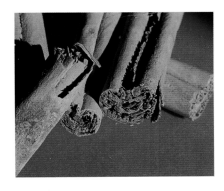

◆ The 'hot' aromatic spices you keep in your kitchen are great for a cold – ginger, cinnamon, cloves, coriander seeds.

◆ Simmer gently for 15 minutes, strain and drink piping hot. Put a cup of red wine in a saucepan and drop in a couple of whole cloves, a pinch of powdered cinnamon, a pinch of powdered ginger and a few crushed coriander seeds.

◆ When you feel all stuffed up use one of nature's nose-clearers. Eucalyptus leaves contain eucalyptol to loosen phlegm. It is antiviral and antimicrobial.

◆ Rub a few drops of essential oil of eucalyptus into the palms of your hands, cup them around your nose and sniff it. This stimulates blood flow to the lungs and helps clear them out.

◆ Make your own inhaler to carry with you. In this way you will get the full benefit of both the menthol and eucalyptus which expensive over-the-counter remedies make so much of.

◆ Fill a small bottle almost to the top with Malden Salt Flakes (see Resources). Add a few drops each of essential oil of eucalyptus and essential oil of peppermint. Shake well. Hold the bottle under your nose and take a good sniff to clear a stuffy head. Keep the lid on when you are not using it.

symptom	what to use	how to use it

Soothing treatments cont.

◆ Goldenrod (*Solidago virgaurea*) soothes mucous membranes. If your nose is sore and dripping, try drinking a cup or two of the tea.

◆ Put 2-3 teaspoons of the dried herb in a tea pot and pour a cup of boiling water over it. Steep for 10 minutes, strain and drink three times a day.

◆ Use daily steam inhalations (see page 188)

◆ Use a few drops of eucalyptus oil, peppermint oil, or lavender oil; a handful of fresh yarrow or elderflowers as they soothe the mucous membranes of your nose. Or put a handful of fresh camomile flowers into a bowl of hot water to calm your nerves.

Sore throat
When a sore throat makes the very act of swallowing an ordeal, reach for soothing herbs to take the sting away.

◆ Sage, hyssop, thyme, goldenseal and marjoram make good, simple gargles to fight infection.

Caution: *Don't use goldenseal if you are pregnant.*

◆ Make a strong infusion of 2 teaspoons of the dried herb to a cup of boiling water and let it steep for 20 minutes. Cool and strain. Gargle with it two to three times a day. For increased power add ½ teaspoon of tincture of echinacea to a cup of the gargle.

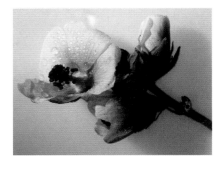

◆ Marshmallow has a high mucilage content. It soothes irritation, eases the pain of a sore throat, and calms inflammation. It is also antiseptic.

◆ Put 1 teaspoon of finely chopped marshmallow root (or a teaspoon of the dried herb) into a tea pot with 300 ml (½ pint) of boiling water. Let stand for half an hour to draw out as much mucilage as possible. Strain and sip throughout the day. Keep any left-over infusion in the fridge and make it fresh every day, it doesn't keep well.

Coughs
Coughs are one of the body's ways of getting rid of whatever bacteria has caused the problem. Rather than try to stop the coughing it is better to help the process along with expectorant herbs that help release phlegm, as well as soothing herbs to ease throat irritation.

◆ Use antimicrobial herbs like eucalyptus, tea tree, thyme and bergamot in a steam inhalation to get right to the problem-causing microbes (see page 188).

Coughs cont.

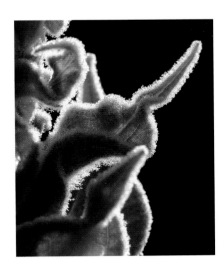

◆ My herb of choice for a tight congested cough is the glorious mullein. You can't miss it. It has grey-green furry leaves and a majestic flower spike covered in creamy yellow flowers that can reach 150 cm (5 ft) in height. It is an excellent expectorant. Combine its anti-inflammatory action and high mucilage content and you will find it soothes even the parts that other herbs can't reach. I also like to mix mullein with anti-microbial and anti-spasmodic thyme, as well as goldenseal. It has a fearsome power to knock out bacteria with a gentle anti-inflammatory effect.

◆ For a chest that aches from too much coughing, make a warming vapour rub.

◆ Liquorice can rescue a chest and throat wracked by a cough. It is anti-inflammatory, antiviral, and soothing thanks to its high mucilage content. It also tastes good.

◆ For a really dry throat use honey in a home-made cough mixture. It is antibacterial and you can make a very simple cough syrup by mixing any infusion or tincture into honey.

◆ I like to use mullein tincture since mullein makes a strong-tasting tea. Take ¼-½ teaspoon of mullein tincture four or five times a day. If you prefer teas to tinctures use, 1-2 teaspoons of the dried leaves or flowers to a cup of boiling water. Steep for 10-15 minutes. Be very careful to strain the tea well as the little hairs on the leaves can actually irritate a sore throat. Mix it with plenty of honey.

◆ Mix together: 2 teaspoons tincture of mullein, ½ teaspoon tincture of thyme and ½ teaspoon tincture of goldenseal. Take ½ teaspoon of this remedy in a little water three times a day.

◆ To ¼ cup almond oil or a small jar of petroleum jelly (Vaseline) add ¼ teaspoon of tincture of mullein and 2 drops each of essential oil of eucalyptus and essential oil of thyme. You may need to gently heat the petroleum jelly in a double boiler to allow the mullein tincture to mix in. Rub into the neck and chest, lie back and let go.

◆ When your throat is dry and sore make a delicious cup of liquorice tea by simmering 1 teaspoon of the chopped root in a cup of water for 20 minutes. Drink it three times a day, but don't over do it as it might cause digestive upset.

◆ The proportions are: 225 g (8 oz) honey to which you add either 225 ml (8 fl oz) infusion or 125 ml (4 fl oz) water and 125 ml (4 fl oz) tincture.

symptom	what to use	how to use it

Coughs cont.

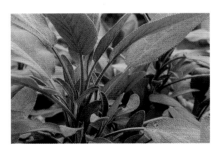

◆ Sage and thyme make a good microbe-fighting cough mixture: use them together or separately. Use tincture of mullein to make an expectorant linctus.

◆ Put 3 tablespoons of the dried, whole leaves into a tea pot. Cover with 475 ml (1 pint) of boiling water, put the lid on and leave it until it has gone cold. Strain, and add 225 ml (8 fl oz) of your infusion to 225 g (8 oz) of honey. Or, add 125 ml (4 fl oz) water and 125 ml (4 fl oz) tincture of sage or thyme to 225 g (8 oz) honey. Take this mixture every hour by the teaspoon.

◆ For a warming cough mixture finely chop an onion.

◆ Put it in a double-boiler with enough honey to cover it and warm it gently for 40 minutes. Strain the mixture. Take it by the teaspoon whenever you need it. It is expectorant and anti-microbial, and it warms deeply.

Caution: *Be sure to use a corked bottle to store them, and keep them somewhere cool. I keep mine in the fridge. Syrups sometimes ferment and there have been one or two nasty explosions in my house when I've used screw-top jars.*

◆ One of my favourite ways to combat a cough is to give it a dose of good wine. This needs to be prepared in advance but it stores well. Any of the herbs mentioned above make a good cough tonic but some taste better than others, so choose one that you enjoy drinking as a tea.

◆ Put 1.2L (2 pints) of good quality white wine into a jar with 100 g (4 oz) dried thyme leaves (or two good handfuls of fresh herb). Tightly screw on the lid and leave the herbs to steep into the wine for two weeks. Strain the herbs out of the wine and rebottle. Sip a glass of tonic wine after your evening meal or just before bed.

Blocked sinuses

◆ The same herbs that are good for congestion in the lungs also help congested sinuses.

◆ Use essential oil of peppermint, eucalyptus, or bergamot to make a steam inhalation (see page 188).
◆ Elderflower tea also helps inflamed sinuses (see page 59).
◆ Drink the chicken soup recommended for colds (see page 188).

symptom	what to use	how to use it
Handling hayfever Dealing with the yearly unwelcome arrival of hayfever demands a two-pronged approach – prevention and easing symptoms that have already appeared. Prevent it early by beginning two months before the hayfever season arrives.	◆ Take tincture of echinacea.	◆ Take 1 teaspoon in a little water three times a day, to build up your immune system.
	◆ Drink nettle tea as it contains small amounts of histamine – the substance that triggers allergies.	◆ Drink nettle tea every day (see page 60) building up to three cups a day.
	◆ All through the winter months take bee pollen each day. This helps build your resistance to airborne pollen six months down the road during hayfever season.	◆ Take 1 teaspoon every morning on an empty stomach.
	◆ Make an infusion of camomile.	◆ Put 1 teaspoon of the dried flowers into a bowl and pour a cup of boiling water over them. Steep for 10 minutes. Soak a piece of cotton in the infusion and allow it to cool. Lie down and place the damp cotton over your eyelids.
Eye relief	◆ Take eyebright (*Euphrasia officinalis*) tincture	◆ Take 1 teaspoon in a little water three times a day when your eyes are itchy. ◆ Put 5 drops of eyebright tincture into a bowl of cold water and use it to gently bathe sore eyes.

hands and feet

Your hands and feet may be the most used and little cared for part of your body. Gentle herbs will soothe them when they're sore and heal them when they develop problems.

symptom	what to use	how to use it

Athlete's foot

Athlete's foot is a tiny fungus that loves warm, moist places. When it has found the perfect place – between your toes, even under nails – it burrows in and makes itself at home. The good news is, athlete's foot hates anti-fungal herbs, so use them liberally and you will soon be free of this irritating condition. There are four I particularly recommend – garlic, tea tree, oregano and lavender, although there are many anti-microbial and anti-fungal herbs that will do the trick. I like these four because I've usually got some in the house. Remember – athlete's foot likes warm, damp places so always dry your feet well and put your towel straight into the laundry basket. And don't reuse it before it's been washed or you will spread the fungus. Wear cotton socks, and wear shoes that let your feet breathe. Avoid those sweaty old trainers.

◆ Garlic is powerfully antiviral – it may be the smell, but athlete's foot rarely hangs around for long when exposed to it. The odd thing about garlic is that even applying it to your feet can make your breath smell, it moves that quickly through your body. If that worries you, then chew on some fresh parsley to neutralize the garlicky smell.

◆ Tea tree is a wonderful antiseptic plant from Australia. It can head off athlete's foot before it really gets a hold.

Caution: *Tea tree oil is poisonous if taken internally so keep it safely out of the reach of children.*

◆ Use garlic oil (see page 75) soaked into a little cotton wool and applied to the affected areas morning and night.
◆ A wonderfully soothing approach is to put enough warm water into a foot bath to cover your feet then crush 4 cloves of garlic into it. Soak your feet for 20 minutes morning and night. If the garlic irritates your feet, stop using it. It may be too strong for you.

◆ Put 5 drops of tea tree oil into a foot bath with enough warm water to cover your feet. Soak your feet at least once every day for 20 minutes. You should see a marked improvement in five days.
◆ You can also use 1 teaspoon of tea tree oil diluted in 1 teaspoon of water or vegetable oil and apply it to affected areas with a little cotton wool. It relieves itching fast.
Use tea tree oil neat on the top of nails affected by a fungus then put a sticking plaster over it – but be careful not to apply it neat to the skin. It is too strong.
◆ You can make a foot bath using tea tree and garlic essential oils. Put 4 drops of each into a foot bath with just enough warm water to cover the feet. Soak your feet for 20 minutes, twice a day. Or add 4 drops of tea tree oil to your foot bath made with warm water and 4 crushed cloves of garlic.

symptom	what to use	how to use it

Athlete's foot cont.

◆ Thyme and lavender are common to most people's gardens. Both have antimicrobial actions. Cider vinegar is astringent and helps to restore the skin's acid mantle. You need to prepare this wash well in advance. Make it if there is someone in your house who frequently suffers from athlete's foot. In the meantime, use one of the above treatments.

◆ For a footbath, take ½ cup each of fresh thyme leaves and fresh lavender flowers and chop them roughly. (You can also use dried herbs, but then put in only half the quantities.) Toss the herbs in a jar and add 2 cups of cider vinegar. Don't use a jar with a metal lid. The metal will react with the acid in the vinegar. Give the mixture a good shake. Store in a cool dark place for two weeks, strain and bottle. Kept somewhere cool and dark this anti-microbial wash will keep for about a year. When you need it, soak a piece of cotton wool in the wash and apply to affected areas two or three times a day.

Corns

Corns are hard little plugs of dead skin that form on feet when they rub inside poorly fitting shoes. Corns can become quite large and painful. If they do, go and see a chiropodist. But our plant friends can help solve the problem if you deal with corns while they are small.

◆ I wonder if we shouldn't just stuff whole cloves of garlic in our socks, so good is it for foot problems.

◆ A more practical solution for corns is to crush a clove of garlic through a garlic press and pile up the mash on a small piece of gauze. Put the garlicky gauze on to the corn and secure it with sticking plasters or a bandage overnight. Repeat until the corn comes off. Bear in mind that the smell of garlic doesn't take long to get from your feet to your mouth so you might want to chew on a few pieces of parsley in the morning to get rid of the smell.

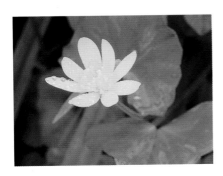

◆ Celandine is one such friend. A beautiful plant that exuberantly tries to take over the lanes around my home in Wales, celandine has glossy golden flowers. The sheer quantity of it makes it my herb of choice during the spring and summer. Of course, wearing shoes that fit properly should stop you getting corns in the first place.

◆ Pick a handful of celandine – flowers, stems and leaves. Crush them or mash them in a mortar until you have a wet paste. Add a little water or vegetable oil if it is too dry. Put the mash on a piece of clean gauze, apply to the corn and bandage in place. Leave on overnight, and keep repeating the process until the corn comes off.

symptom	what to use	how to use it

Verrucas and warts

Warts and verrucas are both caused by viruses. Not so long ago the doctor's treatment of choice was to burn a verruca or wart off the skin. But they found that they soon came back again. You need to kill off the virus to prevent them coming back, which is why herbs work so well. People who are susceptible to warts often have a suppressed immune system. Try taking some of the immune-stimulating herbs mentioned in the chapter on Strengthening, particularly those that are antiviral, such as echinacea and astragalus, to prevent the recurrence of stubborn warts and verrucas.

◆ There are so many folk remedies for warts it's hard to choose. I avoid those that involve burying locks of hair at midnight on a full moon. Here are three remedies that I find highly practical.

◆ Use a garlic poultice, as described on the previous page.

◆ Pick a dandelion flower and rub the milky sap from the stem on to the wart or verruca. The sap creates a sort of crust over the wart or verruca. Continue to apply fresh sap on top of this crust, several times a day. The wart gradually discolours and then comes off. This is a very old folk remedy that relies upon the mysterious milky sap that oozes from the picked flower stem. Dandelion has antiviral properties which, given time, will kill off a wart or verruca.

◆ You need to use a banana that has gone black for this remedy. Take a small part of the blackened peel and place it on your skin with the 'inside' of the peel touching the wart. Put a sticking plaster or piece of gauze around it to hold it in place and leave it on all night. Repeat until the wart has gone.

Chapped hands

Keen herb gardeners will tell you all about the discomfort – and inelegance – of rough, sore, chapped hands. Here are a few quick fixes to put the glamour back into garden hands.

◆ If you have a good, healthy aloe plant that is at least three years old (and you go about it sensibly) you can cut the leaves for use without doing lasting damage to the plant. Relief for sore hands lies inside the leaf.

◆ Cut one, split it open, and smooth the gel you find inside all over your hands.

◆ You can add nourishment to a basic unperfumed hand cream or simple vitamin E cream by mixing in a strong infusion of calendula.

◆ Make your infusion with 8 teaspoons of fresh flower petals (or 4 teaspoons of dried ones) and leave to infuse until the water goes cold. Strain and pour a little at a time into your hand cream. Don't overdo it or you'll end up with milk instead of cream! Smother your hands with your hand cream, leave for 10 minutes, then tissue off the excess.

symptom	what to use	how to use it

Chapped hands cont.

◆ Get gloved. This is just the job for keen gardeners who – even if only rarely – need to present a pair of clean, soft hands to the outside world.

◆ Mix together 2 heaped tablespoons of finely ground almonds (a coffee grinder works well to make them), 1 tablespoon of honey, enough milk (about 2 teaspoons) to make a thick paste, and a couple of drops of essential oil of sandalwood. Cover your hands liberally with the paste and slip them inside disposable plastic gloves (available from any pharmacy). Leave the gloves on overnight. Remove them in the morning and wash your hands in warm water. Repeat for as many nights as you wish to bring your hands back to their former glory.

Head lice

Kids especially can get overrun with head lice. The only things you can get from the chemist to combat them are highly toxic and most unpleasant to use. In particular, there have been cases of toxicity from liberal use of medical pesticidal lotions. Thyme offers a safe and effective alternative. Lice hate it.

◆ Undiluted essential oil of thyme is far too strong to apply neat to skin or scalp.

◆ Instead, add 3-4 drops of the essential oil to a tablespoon of a bland shampoo. Mix well, then massage into wet hair and scalp. Leave for 5 minutes. Rinse thoroughly with warm water. If necessary, you can repeat this thyme shampoo each day for a week to clear the condition.

◆ This part deals with the lice. But their eggs stick to hair shafts and the only way to get rid of them is to loosen the glue that keeps them there. So after shampooing, rinse the hair with equal parts of warm water and cider vinegar. Then wrap the scalp in plastic or a shower cap for 15 minutes. Comb the hair thoroughly with a nit comb dipped in hot vinegar and rinse thoroughly. Repeat the whole process after a week just in case any of the nits remain and hatch.

◆ In the meantime, comb the hair through with the nit comb each day and put a couple of drops of tea tree oil on to the comb just for safe keeping.

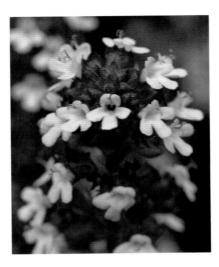

tender tummies

Whether it be constipation or diarrhoea, nausea or hiccoughs, an unsettled stomach robs your day of charm. There are some shining stars among the plants to soothe a disgruntled stomach. Simply taking time over your food can also prevent problems.

symptom	what to use	how to use it
Indigestion If you often have indigestion, it may be the result of poor acid/alkaline balance in the foods you are eating. Avoid too many acid-forming foods such as highly processed convenience foods filled with sugar and junk fats, too much red meat, tomatoes and citrus fruits. Seek medical advice if the problem persists. But for that, 'Oh I wish I hadn't eaten so much' feeling there are a few herbal helpers to give a little instant relief.	◆ Imagine that your stomach is cross with you for giving it more to do than it can manage. You want to make it feel calm and relaxed so it can do its job with ease. ◆ If you have eaten a big meal last thing at night and feel too full to sleep, try a little tincture of valerian. ◆ Try sniffing one of the calming essential oils.	◆ Indian people chew fennel seeds after a meal to aid digestion. It is a good practice. This is one of the reasons I use it in my Herbal Cleanse (see pages 46-8). ◆ Use ½ teaspoon in a little water. Sip it slowly. It can help ease your stomach. ◆ Put a few drops of essential oil of basil, hyssop, rosemary, or lavender in an oil burner or diffuser, or simply put a few drops on a handkerchief and hold it near your nose.
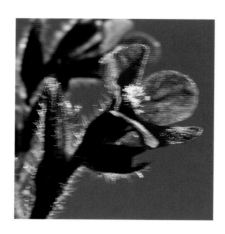	◆ Chocolate manufacturers have made a small fortune out of the after-dinner mint regime. Peppermint is famed for its ability to aid digestion. A cup of peppermint tea will do much more for indigestion than a chocolate. Just the smell rising on its steam works to calm the nerves in your stomach. It will also give a boost to your digestive enzymes, helping them to cope with whatever you have just asked them to deal with. ◆ If you are feeling 'windy' after a meal add a little spice to your tea. This is particularly delicious with fennel tea.	◆ Put 2 teaspoons of dried peppermint leaves or 2 tablespoons of fresh (this is best) into a tea pot and pour a cup of boiling water over them. Allow it to steep for 10 minutes and sip it slowly. Peppermint is one of the herb teas you can easily find in tea bags. Mix it with camomile for added digestive help – use 1 teaspoon of dried peppermint and 1 teaspoon of camomile to a cup of boiling water. ◆ Add a tiny amount (and I mean tiny – the smallest pinch) of cayenne pepper, or a little sprinkling of powdered cinnamon or nutmeg to ease that bloated feeling and prevent embarrassing noises.

Constipation

Constipation means different things to different people. It is almost always an indication of poor eating habits or more serious problems so seek help. Healthy people on a good natural diet will clear their bodies of solid wastes after each meal, not just once a day. For the odd time of increased stress or emotional upset that can cause a sluggish system, increase your intake of raw vegetables and fruits, whole grains such as brown rice, rye and steel-cut oats, and – my favourite – eat stewed rhubarb when in season. If your stomach is still on a go-slow, here are a few ways to get things moving again.

◆ Flax seeds are high in essential fatty acids and fibre. They act as a lubricant on the lower intestine. They also help soothe irritated mucous membranes in the stomach. You can drink this last thing at night if you like.

◆ Sometimes your stomach just needs a little reminder of what it is meant to be doing. The bitter principles in dandelion can often kick-start good digestion.

◆ Reach for liquorice.

Caution: *Don't drink more than two cups a day and for no more than a couple of days. Liquorice packs quite a punch and can cause water retention and digestive upset.*

◆ Take a glass of prune juice mixed with flax seeds for breakfast.
◆ Don't forget to sprinkle flax seeds over your salads too (see also prune juice and flax seeds on page 47).

◆ Add a teaspoon of dandelion root tincture to ½ cup water. Hold each mouthful you take in your mouth for a minute or so to get the benefit of the bitterness. Do this three times a day for a couple of days until the constipation eases. If it doesn't, seek professional help.

◆ Chew a piece of liquorice – the real thing, not the sweets. Or try 1 tablespoon of liquorice root boiled in a cup of water for 30 minutes. This makes a sweet and laxative tea. Strain it and drink.

Diarrhoea

If you often have chronic diarrhoea, you need to seek medical help to find out what is at the root of the problem. It may be something as simple as a change in diet that's needed. But diarrhoea can sometimes be a symptom of more serious conditions so it's as well to check. For that rare, awful attack that lasts no more than a heated 48 hours, here are some emergency measures.

◆ Drink lots. Instinct might tell you that if you stop putting liquids in at one end they will stop coming out at the other. This is not the case. The main danger with diarrhoea is dehydration and you actually need to replenish lost fluids quickly.

◆ Lots of herb tea is perfect, particularly if you choose astringent ones that will help to dry up diarrhoea quickly. Drink green tea, rosemary tea or yarrow tea – 1 teaspoon of the dried herb to a cup of boiling water steeped for 5 minutes should do the trick.

tender tummies

symptom	what to use	how to use it

Diarrhoea cont.

◆ Cinnamon is naturally astringent. It helps dry things up.

◆ Take a cinnamon stick and crush enough of it so you have a tablespoon of crumbled herb. Put it in a tea pot and pour a cup of boiling water over it. Steep for 10-15 minutes and drink it warm and often.

◆ Diarrhoea causes minerals to be lost from the system. Nettle tea is full of minerals to replenish those that have been flushed away.

◆ Collect young, fresh nettle leaves before their stinging hairs have had a chance to form properly. Put 2-4 teaspoons of leaves into a tea pot and pour a cup of boiling water over them. Steep for 10 minutes, strain well and drink.

Nausea

Vomiting is your body's way of getting rid of something it really doesn't want. Suppressing it is not always the best thing to do. But you can feel shaky and uncomfortable during and after a bout of vomiting and there are many herbs that will make you feel much better. It's fine to use ginger when you are pregnant, but avoid using hops, parsley, or, most especially, peppermint when carrying a baby as they may stimulate the uterus.

◆ Sipping ginger tea can relieve nausea quickly and gently. But there are times when you can't keep anything down at all. You can actually absorb enough ginger through your skin to settle your stomach without it having to pass your lips. Use it fresh if you have a root in the fridge. Or use dry powdered ginger root.

◆ Into a bowl of warm water put 1 tablespoon of grated fresh root or 1 tablespoon of powdered ginger (stir it in well). Rest your hands in the ginger water until you feel better. You can also do this in a foot bath.

◆ Alternatively, put 1 tablespoon of fresh grated ginger or 1 tablespoon of powdered ginger into a bath bag (see page 128) or tie it in the middle of a square of muslin – pull up the corners and secure the lot with an elastic band. Run yourself a soothing bath and drop the bag under the taps. Relax in the water for 20 minutes. You should feel much better.

◆ You can also make ginger tea. Grate enough fresh ginger root to fill a tablespoon. Put it into a tea pot and pour a cup of boiling water over it. Sip it ever so slowly. A teaspoon of tincture of ginger in a cup of water sipped slowly will also do the trick.

symptom	what to use	how to use it

Nausea cont.

◆ Just feeling nauseous can be as frightening as vomiting. This is why often just calming yourself eases your stomach and banishes the nausea. These are my favourite soothing herbs.

◆ Meadowsweet tea calms a traumatized system. Use 2 teaspoons of dried herb (flowers and leaves) to a cup of boiling water. Steep for 5-10 minutes. Strain and sip.
◆ Peppermint settles the stomach. It is also powerfully antispasmodic so is especially helpful when you are still trying to vomit even though your stomach is empty (see page 57 for peppermint tea).
◆ Cinnamon contains catechins to help relieve nausea (see opposite for cinnamon tea).
◆ Hops are also rich in catechins. Hop tea is the perfect tea to drink at night or whenever you want to sleep off your nausea. Put 1 teaspoon of the dried flowers into a tea pot with a cup of boiling water and steep for 10 minutes.
◆ Sniff essential oil of peppermint or lavender dropped on to a handkerchief, or put it into an essential oil diffuser and fill the room with its fragrance.

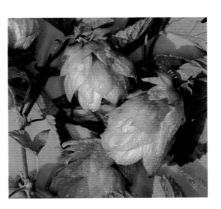

Hiccoughs

Everyone has their favourite hiccough cure. Here is mine. If you have a delicate stomach, however, don't try it. Instead, take a deep breath and drink a big glass of water until you need to breathe again. That should handle the problem.

◆ Take a dessertspoon of cider vinegar – neat. It takes your breath away and seems to shock the system into stopping the hiccoughs. You can also use a teaspoon of herb vinegar made with rosemary.

◆ Put 300 ml (½ pint) of cider vinegar and 300 ml (½ pint) of spring water into a glass jar with 2 tablespoons of fresh rosemary. Put the lid on the jar and leave it in a warm place – an airing cupboard is ideal. Leave it for 10 days, giving it a shake every time you remember it. Strain the vinegar and bottle.

first aid

Having brought up four children I've done my fair share of first aid. I have found the help herbs can offer in an emergency to calm and soothe absolutely invaluable. Here is a collection of the tricks and tips I have picked up along the way. It is also a handy guide to using my First Aid Kit.

symptom	what to use	how to use
Bruises Bruises are broken blood vessels which have leaked blood under the surface of the skin. They often look a lot worse than they really are.	◆ Use arnica ointment – but only if the skin is unbroken (see page 207). ◆ Alternatively, make use of parsley.	◆ Arnica can be toxic if taken internally or absorbed into the blood stream. ◆ Put a couple of handfuls of parsley in a blender with ½ cup water so it makes a green, muddy mess. Pour it into ice-cube trays and freeze. When you have a bruise simply take a green ice cube, wrap it in a tea towel or some muslin and hold it on the bruise. The ice will take away pain and reduce swelling while the parsley helps heal the tissue.
	◆ Or call on comfrey. If you have fresh comfrey growing in your garden, make a comfrey poultice of it. This is great for any kind of bruise or sprain.	◆ Crush a big handful of fresh comfrey leaves (or add several tablespoons of dried comfrey leaves to an equal amount of warm water). Put them between two layers of gauze to hold them together. Place the compress on the bruise and bind it in place with a bandage. Leave it on for at least a couple of hours. When the pain has subsided apply calendula and comfrey ointment (see page 34) to further speed the healing process.
Burns Most burns are minor and caused by carelessness around the home. A serious burn needs to be dealt with quickly by a hospital. For a minor scald – a slip in the oven, or a close encounter with the iron – a little emergency first aid works wonders.	◆ Cool the burn immediately by running cold water over it for at least 10 minutes to take the heat out of it. Then apply some aloe gel or calendula to increase blood flow to the burnt area to help it to heal more quickly.	◆ Smooth it over the burn where it will take away the pain, reduce swelling and keep the skin moist. Or you can just slit the leaf, open it up and lay the gel side on the burn. Hold it in place with a bandage.

symptom	what to use	how to use

Burns cont.

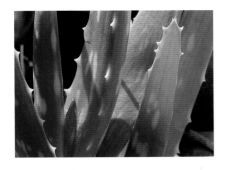

◆ If you don't have an aloe plant, then cool the burn and pat on a little St John's wort oil.

◆ Drink a cup of willow bark tea to ease pain, and take a little Rescue Remedy.

◆ When the burn is healing apply calendula and comfrey ointment to reduce scarring. Don't use it on deep burns, however, or any that appear to be infected. These two herbs are so strong in their action that they can spur the skin to heal so quickly on the surface that infection gets trapped beneath, or so deeper areas of the wound are unable to heal well.

◆ See First Aid Kit on page 208. Reapply the oil three times a day until the burn has healed. This helps take away the pain and reduces scarring.

◆ For willow bark tea, see recipe on page 208. For Rescue Remedy, see First Aid Kit on page 208.

◆ See recipe on page 34.

Cuts and scrapes

A little help is all your body needs to do an excellent repair job on minor cuts and scrapes. Clean up the wound, encourage the natural healing process and let nature do the rest.

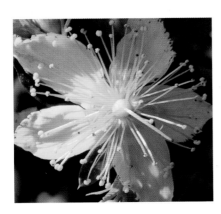

◆ Wash the cut or scrape well with clean water. Then bathe with tea tree or manuka essential oil.

◆ Or if you have tinctures of echinacea, calendula and St John's wort you can make an alternative antiseptic wound wash.

◆ Apply a little St John's wort oil to take the sting out of any minor wound.

◆ After a day or two apply calendula and comfrey ointment to speed healing and lessen scarring.

◆ If, however, it looks like infection is setting in, use an echinacea wash.

◆ Use 4 drops oil to ½ cup water. Soak cotton wool and wipe over the cut or scrape to prevent infection.

◆ Put 2 teaspoons of each tincture into a dark glass bottle and keep in the fridge. When you need it, use 2 teaspoons of the mixture in 2 teaspoons of clean water and swab the wound with it.

◆ See First Aid Kit on page 208.

◆ See recipe on page 34.

◆ Mix 1 teaspoon of tincture to 3 teaspoons water. Apply every two hours.

symptom	what to use	how to use

Cuts and scrapes cont.

◆ If you have fallen foul of a sharp kitchen knife, reach for the spice rack.

◆ A tiny amount of cayenne pepper helps stop bleeding, and a little powdered cloves helps stave off infection. Rescue Remedy will deal with the shock.

◆ Whenever you are out and about and get cut, use fresh yarrow leaves.

◆ Press them to any cuts or scrapes to stop bleeding and speed healing.

Insect bites and stings

Insect bites and stings are little more than a painful irritation. If you are stung by something large like a bee or wasp (always remove the sting as quickly as you can) and have difficulty breathing or develop a rash, make your way to hospital quickly; a few people have severe allergic reactions to them. See your doctor, too, if a bite or sting becomes infected or you feel feverish or unwell.

◆ Use peppermint oil. It is antiseptic and pain killing. Wash your hands after using it as it can play havoc if you get it in your eyes.

◆ Put a drop right in the middle of any bite or sting and it will stop the itching.

◆ Alternatively, try a drop of lavender oil.

◆ Put it on the bite or sting will soothe. It is particularly good for mosquito bites.

◆ Use tincture of echinacea externally or internally.

◆ Bathe the bite or sting every hour with 1 teaspoon of tincture of echinacea to 1 teaspoon of water. You can also take it internally to help prevent infection – 1 teaspoon in water three times a day (not for children).

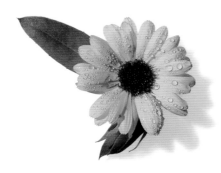

◆ The next day apply calendula and comfrey ointment to the area.

◆ See recipe on page 34.

◆ When you are out in nature and get stung, grab a handful of chickweed.

◆ Rub it between your hands to release the juices and press the mush to the sting. Keep it on until it begins to dry out then repeat the process.

◆ Old folk remedies often help a lot. Try applying honey to bee stings and lemon juice to wasp stings.

symptom	what to use	how to use
Splinters	◆ You can use leftover flax seeds from The Herbal Cleanse (see page 46) to draw out hard-to-handle deep splinters.	◆ Grind 1 teaspoon of flax seeds in your coffee grinder. Mix with just enough water to make a thick paste. Pile on top of the splinter and cover with a bandage. Replace every day. It should take no more than a week to work its way out.
	◆ Follow with an application of calendula and comfrey ointment.	◆ See recipe on page 34.
Sprains and strains Strains happen to muscles, sprains to joints. They happen when you force the muscle or joint to move further than is natural for it. Seek medical help if you are in severe pain, you may find you have broken a bone.	◆ The first course of action is to place an ice pack on the injury to reduce the swelling. A packet of frozen peas works well. As they warm up you can refreeze them and then reapply. Then drink a cup of willow bark tea to ease pain, and take Rescue Remedy for the shock.	◆ For willow bark tea see recipe on page 208. For Rescue Remedy see First Aid Kit, page 208.
	◆ Use essential oil of thyme. Thyme is antispasmodic and stimulates blood flow to the injury so speeding healing.	◆ Add 10 drops to 2 cups of cold water and use as a compress. Soak a length of cotton sheet or bandage in the mixture and wring it out. Fold the cloth so that it covers the injured part and loosely bind the compress on with a cotton bandage. Alternate 2 minutes of compress with 2 minutes of ice pack, or if this is disturbing the injury too much, leave the compress on and cover it with the ice pack.
	◆ You can use a compress of cayenne pepper in the same way if you have some to hand.	◆ Make an infusion of ½ teaspoon of cayenne in 1 cup of boiling water. Steep for just a few minutes. Take a tablespoon of the infusion and add it to a cup of hot water to dilute it. Soak a cotton bandage in it and make a compress as with thyme. If the cayenne burns your skin, stop immediately and wash the area well.

symptom	what to use	how to use
Sprains and strains cont.	◆ Apply arnica ointment, St John's wort oil, or calendula and comfrey ointment to ease the pain and help with the healing.	◆ See First Aid Kit on page 208, and for calendula and comfrey ointment see recipe on page 34.
	◆ When the sprain or strain is on the mend, mix essential oils of thyme and lavender.	◆ Mix 5 drops of essential oil of thyme with 5 drops of essential oil of lavender in a tablespoon of carrier oil (almond or olive). Use as a massage oil to soothe and help with the blood flow and healing. If it's painful, stop doing the massage. Try again in a few days.
Sunburn Even using sunblock the sun can catch you out and you get fried. If the skin blisters, you feel unwell, or go hot and cold, seek medical attention. Minor sunburn you can deal with at home.	◆ Take a cool bath to with added ingredients.	◆ Add 2 to 3 drops of lavender oil for soothing plus 1 tablespoon of cider vinegar to restore the skin's natural acid mantle.
	◆ Use aloe vera immediately as you would for any burn.	◆ Smooth the gel straight from the leaf or the tube on the skin, but don't rub it in.
	◆ Make a cooling spray.	◆ Put a few drops of lavender essential oil in a plant spray bottle with 100 g (4 oz) aloe vera juice – not gel – and 300 ml (½ pint) water. Shake well and spray liberally over the area.

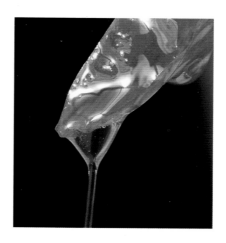

the first aid kit

I believe in simplicity. Why have a first aid kit so full of creams, oils, pills and potions that you can't remember what to do with them? My own has the bare essentials so when it is needed, it swings into action immediately. It is easy to put together your own kit. You need to buy a few essential oils. The rest of the kit you can either buy or make at home, whichever is easiest for you.

remedy	what it does	how to use
Arnica ointment for bruises and sprains (make or buy)	◆ Contains anti-inflammatory helenalin, provides pain relief, is antiseptic and anti-inflammatory.	◆ Rub it on bruises and bumps, sprains and strains. Apply ice to the injury first to reduce the swelling and follow with your arnica cream. Repeat twice a day until healed. Caution: *Do not use arnica on broken skin and never take internally. It is a poison.*
Aloe vera gel – better still an aloe vera plant (make or buy)	◆ For burns and healing skin aloe vera gel is soothing, antiseptic and anti-inflammatory if only extracted from the leaf pulp. It contains carboxypeptidase and bradykininase which relieve pain. It will help soothe burns, including sunburn.	◆ Apply to minor burns and sunburn. Cut a leaf of the plant or use proprietary aloe vera gel. Smooth the gel over the burn. It will help take away the pain, reduce swelling and keep the skin moist to allow graceful healing. ◆ If you have a plant, pick a leaf, slit it open and use the gel fresh. Or slit open a leaf and lay the gel side on the burn. Hold it in place with a bandage.
Calendula and comfrey ointment or cream (make or buy)	◆ For cuts, scrapes and bruises, comfrey contains allantoin to speed skin healing. Calendula contains triterpenes, which encourage new cell growth.	◆ Apply the ointment or cream to bumps and bruises as an alternative to arnica ointment (see above). ◆ Wash cuts and scrapes first with diluted tea tree oil (see overleaf) then apply calendula and comfrey ointment. ◆ Use it on burns once they have begun to heal to reduce scarring. Do not apply to fresh burns.

remedy	what it does	how to use
St John's wort oil (make or buy)	◆ For sunburn, strains, insect bites and stings, hypericum oil brings pain relief when you apply it to skin. Do not use internally.	◆ Use the oil (see page 34) on clean minor burns and sunburn as well as to relieve pain. Apply it to strains and sprains, after the injury has been cooled with ice to reduce swelling. ◆ Put it on insect bites and stings (ensuring the stings have been removed) to relieve pain and itching. Caution: *Do not take St John's wort oil internally.*
Tea tree oil or manuka oil (to buy)	◆ Tea tree contains the powerful antiseptic terpinen-4-ol. Do not use internally.	◆ Dilute 4 drops of essential oil of tea tree or manuka oil in ½ cup of water to make an antiseptic wash for cuts and scrapes. Wash wounds well with clean water, then soak a piece of cotton wool in tea tree and water and swab the wound to prevent infection.
Willow bark (to buy)	◆ Willow bark contains anti-inflammatory and analgesic plant chemicals to relieve pain and reduce heat.	◆ Make as a tea to relieve pain – pour a cup of boiling water over 1 teaspoon of crushed bark, steep for 15 minutes, strain and drink. Good for injuries such as strains and sprains, and will relieve pain from minor burns and sunburn.
Tincture of echinacea (to buy)	◆ An internal antiseptic. Although you can make your own tincture I would recommend buying some from a reputable supplier to ensure a good level of active constituents.	◆ Take 1 teaspoon of tincture in a little water 3 times a day where there is risk of infection from cuts and scrapes, burns and sunburn.
Rescue Remedy (to buy)	◆ Dr Bach's famous flower remedy. A few drops sipped from a glass of water treats shock	◆ Any injury or emergency – for the patient and the carer! Put a few drops in a glass of water and sip.

remedy	what it does	how to use
Essential oil of peppermint (to buy)	◆ Provides pain relief and is antiseptic for insect bites and stings. Do not use internally.	◆ Use a drop of the oil neat on insect bites and stings to relieve pain and itching.
Essential oil of thyme (to buy)	◆ Anti-inflammatory and anti-spasmodic, thyme eases pain. Do not use internally.	◆ Use a compress to relieve sprains and strains. Add 10 drops of the essential oil to 4 tablespoons of cold water. Soak a length of cotton sheet in the mixture and wring it out. Fold the cloth so that it covers the injured part and loosely bind with a cotton bandage. Alternate ice pack and compress every 2 minutes.
Essential oil of lavender (to buy) 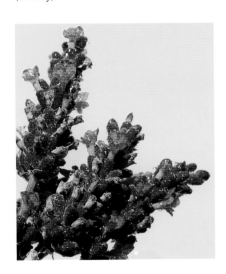	◆ Provides pain relief, and is relaxing and soothing. Do not use internally.	◆ A drop of the oil neat on insect bites and stings will soothe pain. ◆ For a headache put one drop behind each ear, at the back of the head at the base of the skull on each side, and on each temple (keep your hands and the oil well away from your eyes). ◆ For sunburn, take a cool bath with 2-3 drops of lavender oil to soothe and a tablespoon of cider vinegar to restore the skin's natural acid mantle. Caution: *Do not use any essential oil internally. They can be poisonous.*

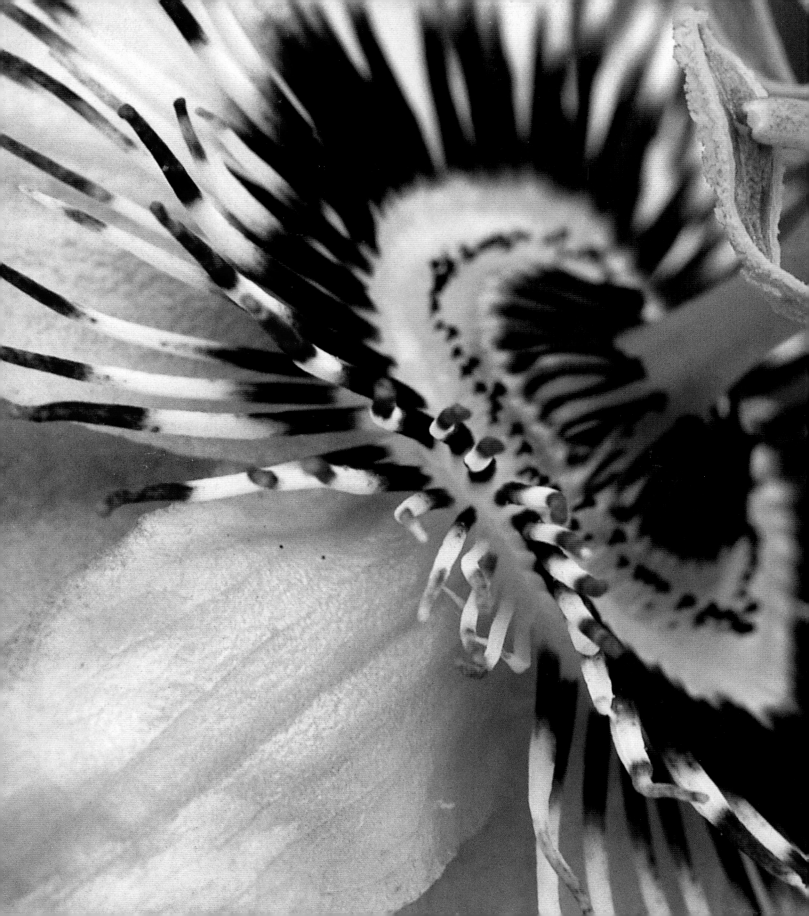

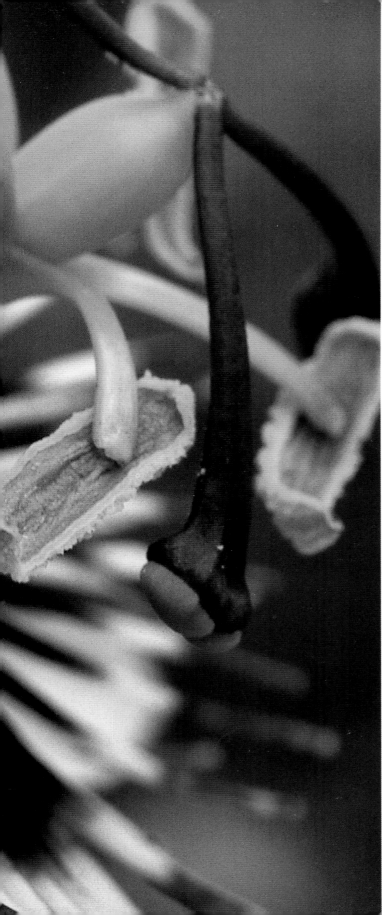

learn more

To glean a deep understanding of herbs is a lifelong quest. Enhance your knowledge by looking further into the actions of herbs (given overleaf) and combine it with a hands-on experience that can only be gleaned by putting herbs into practice. For this a list of Resources is given on pages 215-18 and the Further Reading section outlines many other people's opinions and research.

◄ passionflower

herbs in action

There are many words which professionals use to describe the actions of herbs. Some seem to have come straight out of a medieval manuscript. Don't be put off by them. A lot are self-explanatory – like 'anti catarrhal', 'anti-inflammatory', 'sedative' and 'stimulant'. Others take a little working out. It is worthwhile learning the jargon. Then when you pick up any herbal to check out a plant's action you will know what it's talking about. Here are some of the most common actions of herbs, what they mean and some of the plants that carry each characteristic.

reaction name	meaning	examples of herbs
Alterative	◆ Plants that alter metabolism to improve function. Many are the old-fashioned 'blood cleansers' given for infection. The detoxifiers and balancers, they help to eliminate unwanted material from the whole system and restore order.	◆ Burdock, cleavers, echinacea, garlic, goldenseal, nettle, yellow dock.
Anodyne	◆ These are the pain relievers, the analgesics, those that make pain easier to bear rather than blocking it completely.	◆ Hops, passionflower, St John's wort, skullcap, valerian.
Anthelmintic/vermicide & vermifuge	◆ These herbs kill and expel parasitic worms from the digestive system.	◆ Aloe, garlic, rue, tansy, wormwood.
Anti-emetic	◆ These work to reduce nausea.	◆ Cloves, dill, fennel, ginger, lavender, meadowsweet.
Antiseptic	◆ Most antiseptic herbs do not work to kill off all germs, they make the body a less desirable place for unwanted organisms to settle. They help to keep the body's micro-populations in balance.	◆ Calendula, camomile, garlic, ginger, manuka, rosemary, tea tree, thyme.
Astringent	◆ These herbs precipitate protein – tightening and binding tissue. They are used for conditions such as haemorrhage and diarrhoea and for skincare to tone the skin. Astringent herbs that stop bleeding to external wounds are called 'styptic'.	◆ Eyebright, goldenrod, meadowsweet, mullein, plantain, raspberry, red sage, rosemary, St John's wort, yarrow.

reaction name	meaning	examples of herbs
Bitter	◆ These are herbs that taste bitter and so have a reflex action as a tonic for the digestive system. Generally it is necessary to taste the bitter flavours for the reflex to work.	◆ Blessed thistle, camomile, dandelion root, goldenseal, hops, mugwort, rue, southernwood, wormwood, yarrow.
Carminative	◆ These herbs calm the stomach and aid the release of gas. They work by improving blood supply and 'warming' the stomach.	◆ Angelica, camomile, cardamom, cinnamon, dill, fennel, garlic, ginger, hyssop, mustard, peppermint, sage, thyme, valerian.
Demulcent	◆ These herbs comfort and soothe internal soft tissue such as the digestive tract, liver and kidneys. They can also relieve irritation of the skin and provide a moisturizing, protective coating.	◆ Comfrey, flax seed, liquorice, marshmallow, mullein, slippery elm.
Diaphoretic	◆ These are also herbs for detoxification. They specifically help elimination through the skin as they produce sweat and are particularly useful in treating fever.	◆ Angelica, black cohosh, camomile, elder, fennel, garlic, ginger, golden rod, peppermint, thyme, yarrow.
Diuretic	◆ These herbs increase urine production and so help with elimination. Many are high in potassium so there is no potassium loss when using them as with prescription diuretics.	◆ Burdock, cleavers, dandelion, elder, hawthorn berries, parsley, saw palmetto, wild carrot, yarrow.
Emmenagogue	◆ These herbs aid the female reproductive system, promoting normal menstrual flow. The term can also be used to mean herbs that act as tonics to the female reproductive system.	◆ Black cohosh, black haw, calendula, camomile, chastetree, false unicorn root, fenugreek, ginger, goldenseal, motherwort, parsley, peppermint, raspberry, red sage, rosemary, rue, St John's wort, southernwood, thyme, valerian, yarrow.
Emollient	◆ These herbs soften or soothe the skin due to their high mucilage (gelatinous) constituents. They have a gluey stickiness.	◆ Borage, comfrey, fenugreek, flax seed, liquorice, marshmallow, mullein, rose petals, slippery elm.

herbs in action cont.

reaction name	meaning	examples of herbs
Expectorant	◆ These herbs help the body to get rid of excess mucus from the lungs and respiratory system, especially after a cold or flu.	◆ Angelica, blessed thistle, borage, calendula, cayenne, elderflower, Comfrey, elderflower, garlic, goldenseal, hyssop, liquorice, marshmallow, mullein, thyme, vervain.
Febrifuge	◆ These herbs help to bring down a fever. This classification is often used to include diaphoretic herbs.	◆ Eucalyptus, hyssop, peppermint, raspberry, red sage, thyme, vervain.
Hepatic	◆ These herbs are used to strengthen the liver.	◆ Aloe, dandelion root, fennel, goldenseal, hyssop, motherwort, wild yam, wormwood, yarrow, yellow dock.
Hypnotic	◆ I include this one because people think if you take a hypnotic herb you will fall into a trance. Not so. Hypnotics simply encourage sleep.	◆ Hops, passionflower, skullcap, valerian, wild lettuce.
Nervine	◆ These herbs balance the nervous system, allowing it to cope well with stress without using up too much nervous energy.	◆ Black cohosh, black haw, camomile, ginseng, hops, lavender, motherwort, passionflower, peppermint, rosemary, skullcap, thyme, valerian, vervain, wormwood.
Rubefacient	◆ These herbs are used externally to increase blood circulation in the area to which they are applied. Drawing blood to the surface in this way creates heat and can be used to ease muscular and joint pains and aid decongestion.	◆ Cayenne, cloves, garlic, ginger, mustard, nettle, peppermint oil, rosemary oil, rue.
Vulnerary	◆ These herbs are for the healing of wounds, sprains and bruises. They seal blood leaks from the veins and disperse the fluid that causes swelling. Some also promote healing through cell regeneration.	◆ Aloe, arnica, burdock, calendula, chickweed, comfrey, elder, fenugreek, flax seed, garlic, goldenseal, horsetail, hyssop, marshmallow, mullein, myrrh, St John's wort, slippery elm, thyme, yarrow.

resources

Leslie lectures and teaches workshops throughout the world on health, authentic power, energy, creativity, shamanism, and spirituality. There are two companies who organise workshops for her in Britain: Bright Ideas provides workshops on health, energy and personal empowerment. They also book Leslie for lectures and individually tailored seminars when these are requested. For further information contact Bright Ideas: Telephone (in the UK) 08700 783783, or email LK@bright-idea.

co.uk. The Sacred Trust organizes Leslie's residential and non-residential workshops on freedom, spirituality, creativity, and shamanism. For further information contact The Sacred Trust, PO Box 603, Bath, BA1 2ZU: Telephone 01225 852615, Fax 01225 858961.

Leslie's audio tapes including *10 Steps to a New You*, as well as her videos including *10 Day Clean Up Plan*, *Ageless Ageing*, *Lean Revolution*, *10 Day De-Stress Plan*, and *Cellulite Revolution*, can be ordered

from QED Recording Services Ltd, Lancaster Road, New Barnet, Hertfordshire, EN4 8AS. Telephone 020 8441 7722, Fax 020 8441 0777. Email QED@globalnet.co.uk.

If you want to know about Leslie's personal appearances, forthcoming books, videos, workshops and projects please visit her website for worldwide information: www.qed-productions/lesliekenton.htm. You can also write to her care of QED at the above address enclosing a stamped, self-addressed A4-sized envelope.

herbalists

For information on how to find a good herbalist near to you contact:

GREAT BRITAIN
The General Council & Register of Consultant Herbalists
Marlborough House
Swanpool, Falmouth
Cornwall TR11 4HW
National Institute of Medical Herbalists
56 Longbrook Street
Exeter
Devon EX4 6AH
The National Institute of Herbal Medicine
9 Palace Gate
Exeter
Devon EX1 1JA
British Herbal Medicine Association
Field House
Lyle Hole Lane
Redhill
Avon BS18 7TB
Register of Chinese Herbal Medicine
98b Hazelville Road
London N19 3NA

AUSTRALIA
Herb Society of Western Australia
149 Bradford Street
Coolbinia
Western Australia 6050
Telephone (09) 444 5328
National Herbalist's Association of Australia
PO Box 65
Kingsgrove
NSW 2208
Telephone (02) 787 4523
NEW ZEALAND
The College of Naturopathic Medicine
Box 4529
Christchurch
USA
The American Herbalist Guild
PO Box 1683
Soquel
CA 95073
American Herb Association
Box 353
Rescue
CA 96672
International Herb Growers & Marketers Association
Box 281

Silver Springs
PA 17575
CANADA
The Ontario Herbalists Association
181 Brookdale Avenue
Toronto
Ontario M5M 1P4

herb suppliers

Phyto Products Ltd
Park Works
Park House
Mansfield Woodhouse
Notts NG19 8EF
Telephone 01623 644 334
Fax 01623 657 232
An excellent company originally set up to supply herbalists with high-quality herbs and plant products. Every plant and herb they sell states the source of origin. All Phyto Products' plants are purchased only from recognizable sources. They do a full range of tinctures, herbal skin creams (including Calendula Cream, Comfrey Cream, Arnica Ointment and St John's Wort Oil), fluid extracts, herbs and the Schoenenberger plant juices. Virtually all

the herbs mentioned in this book are supplied by this company in both tincture form and the loose dried herb. They do not supply herbs in capsules but they now do some herbs in tablet form. Write to them for their price list. They have a minimum order of £20 (before VAT) plus carriage.

Weleda (UK) Ltd

Heanor Road
Ilkeston
Derbyshire DE7 8DR
Telephone 0115 944 8200
Fax 0115 944 8210
http//www.weleda.co.uk
Weleda grew out of the work of Rudolf Steiner and have been making medicines and body-care products for 75 years. Weleda UK grow over 400 species of plants organically and biodynamically for use in their medicines and body-care range. They do an excellent arnica cream and a delightful skin-care range. Available from good health stores and pharmacies. Or order direct on 0115 944 8222.

Simmonds Herbal Supplies

Freepost (BR1396)
Hove
West Sussex BN3 6BR
Telephone 01273 202 401
Fax 01273 705 120
Email sales@herbalsupplies.com
This company has been supplying high-quality additive-free 'biodynamic' herbal aids to health practitioners in the UK and abroad since 1982. They now do a range of good-quality products for the general public as well, offering single herbs and mixtures as capsules, tinctures or extracts. Their formula 'Leslie Kenton's Herbal Cleanse' is a mixture of dandelion, burdock and cleavers designed for the Herbal Cleanse on pages 40-51. Order it from them either in capsule or extract form. Write to them for their catalogue.

Bioforce (UK) Ltd

2 Brewster Place
Irvine
Ayrshire
Telephone 01563 851 177
Fax 01563 851 173
Suppliers of herbal extracts, tinctures, homeopathic remedies and natural self-care products and foods, Bioforce is a Swiss company started by the Swiss expert in natural health Alfred Vogel. The company always use fresh herbs in preparing their products at the Bioforce factory in Roggwil. They make over 100 different herbal and homeopathic preparations, all of which are very high quality. They can be ordered by post but are often also available in good health-food stores and pharmacies carrying herbal products.

Bio-Health Ltd

Culpepper Close
Medway City Estate
Rochester
Kent ME2 4HU
Telephone 01483 570813
Bio-Health do an excellent range of single herbs, ointments and multi-herb compounds in tablet and capsule form which you can purchase from good health food-stores or order by post. Write to them for a catalogue.

Solgar Vitamins

Solgar House
Aldbury
Tring
Herts HP23 5PT
Telephone 01442 890 355,
Fax 01442 890 366
An American company founded in 1947 which produces good-quality nutritional supplements and standardized single herbs and formulas under strict pharmaceutical standards of manufacture – in many cases stricter than USA government

requirements. These include standardized full potency Herbal Female Complex (containing soya isoflavones), Feverfew Willow Complex, Milk Thistle Dandelion Complex, Ginger Fennel Complex, Olive Leaf Echinacea Complex and Herbal Male Complex. Solgar products are available from top health-food stores, some chemists and the Nutri Centre.

The Nutri Centre

7 Park Crescent
London W1N 3HE
Telephone 020 7436 5122
Fax 020 7436 5171
The Nutri Centre is on the lower ground floor of the Hale Clinic in London and has the finest selection of nutritional products and books on health under one roof in Britain. It is also able to supply herbs, homeopathic products, Ayurvedic and biochemic products, flower remedies, essential oils, skin-care and dental products, and has an extensive selection of books, including Leslie Kenton's, all available through a good mail-order service.

BioCare Ltd

The Lakeside Centre
180 Liffard Lane
Kings Norton
Birmingham
West Midlands B30 3NU
Telephone 0121 433 3727
Fax 0121 433 3879
A science-based manufacturer of innovative nutritional and health-care products, BioCare was founded nearly 20 years ago by practitioners for practitioners. BioCare products are now available to the public mail order (ring for a catalogue) as well as through suppliers of sophisticated nutritional products such as the Nutri Centre (see above). Their oil-based products, from Vitamin E to Linseed Oil, are all specially formulated to protect

from oxidation by flushing each capsule with nitrogen. In the case of light-sensitive products, BioCare use opaque capsules. They even do chemical-free vitamins in liquid form which have been specially emulsified or micelized to enhance the absorption to 95%. These can be added to juice or water or taken sub-lingually. They are excellent for allergic people or people with digestive problems. BioCare produce the very highest quality nutritional products in Britain.

Higher Nature Ltd
The Nutrition Centre
Burwash Common
East Sussex N19 7LX
Telephone 01435 882 880
Fax 01435 883 720
Higher Nature do a small range of first-rate nutritional supplements which you can order direct, including aloe vera capsules and juice, elderberry extract, flaxseed oil, organic linseeds, stevia, St John's wort, and Soyagen. Write to them for a catalogue.

Xynergy Products
Lower Elstead
Midhurst
West Sussex
GU29 0JT
Telephone 01730 813 642
This company specializes in selling the finest aloe vera products and green nutritional products – such as spirulina and cereal grasses – you can buy. They are available in sophisticated health-food stores or can be ordered by post direct from them.

Neal's Yard Remedies
15 Neal's Yard
Covent Garden
London WC2H 9DP
Telephone 020 7379 722
Mail Order 0161 831 7875
Supply dried herbs, essential oils,

ingredients for making your own remedies and cosmetics, along with books and literature. They also have stores in Oxford, Bromley, Manchester, Bristol and Norwich.

miscellaneous

COSMETICS INGREDIENTS
Available by mail order from **Neal's Yard Remedies** (see above).

ESSENTIAL OILS
Top quality aromatherapy products are available from:**Sandra Day**
Ashley House
185A Drake Street
Rochdale
Lancashire OL11 1E7
Telephone 01706 750302
Fax 01706 750 304

The Fragrant Earth Co Ltd
PO Box 182
Taunton
Somerset, TA1 1YR
Telephone 01823 335 734
Fax 01823 322 566

Purple Flame
Clinton Lane
Kenilworth
Warwickshire CV8 1AS
Telephone 01926 855 980
Fax 01926 512 001

Essentially Oils Ltd
8,9,10, Mount Farm
Junction Road
Churchill
Chipping Norton
Oxfordshire OX7 6NP
Telephone 01608 659 544
Fax 01608 659 522
Also do good-quality oils.

Tisserand Aromatherapy
Newtown Road
Hove
Sussex BN3 7BA
Telephone 01273 325 666

Do an essential oil diffuser that plugs in and fans the oils into the air.

FLAX SEEDS/LINSEEDS
'Linusit Gold' linseeds are available from the Nutri Centre (see above). Organic linseeds are also available from Higher Nature (see above). Keep them refrigerated.

GINSENG
A good ginseng comes in the form of Jinlin Ginseng Tea, Jinlin Panax ginseng dried slices, ampoules and Jinlin whole root, available from health-food stores. They also do ginseng tea in bags and in instant granulated sachets which I use regularly. If you have difficulty finding it contact:

Alice Chiu
4 Tring Close
Barkingside
Essex IG2 7LQ
Telephone 020 8550 9900
Fax 020 8554 3883

HONEY
The New Zealand Natural Food Company have a fine range of honey, including organic honey, in particular Manuka honey, known for its anti-bacterial effects.

The New Zealand Natural Food Company Ltd
Unit 3
55-57 Park Royal Road
London, NW10 7LP
Telephone 020 8961 4410
Fax 020 8961 9420

Evernat
Do a good organic honey from Argentina, available from Planet Organic and good health-food stores. For stockists call 01932 354 211.

INCENSE INGREDIENTS
Powdered charcoal is available from chemists or pharmacies and from any supplier of products for churches. Frankincense, myrrh and benxoin gum are

available from Phyto Products (see page 215). Gum Arabic is available from art suppliers and craft shops.

MALDEN SALT FLAKES

Available from good health-food stores and some supermarkets. This is the best-tasting salt I have ever found. It is spiky and delicious to crumble.

MARIGOLD SWISS VEGETABLE BOUILLON POWDER

This instant broth made from vegetables and sea salt comes in regular, low-salt, vegan and organic varieties. It is available from health-food stores, or direct from:

Marigold Foods

102 Camley Street

London, NW1 0PF

Telephone 020 7388 4515

Fax 020 7388 4516

OLIVE LEAF EXTRACT

Made by Solgar (see page 216) and available from the Nutri Centre (see page 216).

ORGANIC FOODS

The Soil Association publishes a regularly updated National Directory of Farm Shops and Box Schemes which costs £3 including postage from The Organic Food & Farming Centre, 86 Colston Street, Bristol, BS1 5BB. Excellent organic beef, lamb, port, bacon, ham, chicken and sausage, can be ordered from:

Longwood Farm Organic Meats

Tudenham St Mary

Bury St Edmunds

Suffolk IP28 6TB

Telephone 01638 717 120

Organics Direct

Offers a nationwide home delivery service of fresh vegetables and fruits, delicious breads, juices, sprouts, fresh soups, ready-made meals, snacks and baby foods. They also sell the state-of-the-art 2001 Champion Juicer and the 2002 Health Smart Juice Extractor for beginners. They

even sell organic wines – all shipped to you within 24 hours.

Telephone 020 7729 2828

Website: www.organicsdirect.com

You can also order online.

Pure Mail Order

Do organic foods and natural remedies as well as macrobiotic foods mail order. They do herb teas, organic grains, whole seeds for spouting, dried fruits, pulses, nut butters, soya and vegetable products, sea vegetables, drinks and Bioforce herb tinctures. Write to them for a catalogue. You can order by telephone, fax or post.

Pure Multi-Nutrients

6 Victory Place

Crystal Palace

London SE19 3RW

Telephone 020 8771 4522

Fax 020 8771 4522

RESCUE REMEDY

Available from good health-food stores or the Nutri Centre (see page 216) from the range of Bach Flower Remedies.

TEA TREE OIL AND MANUKA OIL

Available from good health-food stores or the Nutri Centre (see page 216).

UDO'S CHOICE

A balance of both Omega 3 and Omega 6 essential fatty acids as well as other important fatty acids such as GLA. Available from good health-food stores or by post from the Nutri Centre (see page 216). Keep refrigerated and do not heat.

FOR INFORMATION ON HERB GROWING, EVENTS, AND GARDENS TO VISIT CONTACT:

The Herb Society

134 Buckingham Palace Road

London SW11 4RW

Telephone 020 7823 5583

The British Herb Growers Association

C/o NFU

Agriculture House

London SW1X 7NJ

useful websites

www.herbs.org

Sells information packs on specific herbs.

www.sympatico.ca/healthyway

A site that provides information and reviews other health sites.

www.all-natural.com/herbindx.html

Contains herbalist Michael Moore's eight clinical herb manuals.

www.thriveonline.com

Provides some of the latest health news, both conventional and alternative.

www.onhealth.com

Alternative and conventional health information, including information on herbs and remedies.

www.yahoo.com/Health/Alternative_ Medicine/Herbs

This site puts you in touch with phytochemical, ethnobotanical and nutritional databases plus access to a comprehensive dictionary of plants and herbs.

www.med.harvard.edu/chge

The Centre for Health and the Global Environment at Harvard Medical School, Boston. This site looks at the relationship of human health to the health of the global environment.

www.headaches.org

Created by the National Headache Foundation, this is a valuable resource for headache sufferers.

further reading

American Herbalist Guild, *American Herbalism: Essay on Herbs and Herbalism*, Freedom, Crossing Press, 1992.

Bacon, Richard M., *The Forgotten Arts. Growing Gardening and Cooking with Herbs*, H.H. Yankee Books, Dublin, 1972.

Beanfield, Harriet & Korngold, *Between Heaven and Earth: A Guide to Chinese Medicine*, Ballantine Books, New York, 1991.

Boxer, Arabella, and Back, Phillipa, *The Herb Book*, Octopus, London, 1980.

Brownlow, Margaret, *Herbs and the Fragrant Garden*, Darton, Longman and Todd, London, 1963.

Campion, K., *A Woman's Herbal*, Vermilion, London, UK, 1992.

Castleman, Michael, *The Healing Herbs: The Ultimate Guide to the Curative Powers of Nature's Medicines*, Emmaus, Rodale Press, 1991.

Chancellor, P., *Illustrated Handbook of Bach Flower Remedies*, The C. W. Daniels Co. Ltd., London, UK, 1971.

Christoper, Dr John R., *School of Natural Healing*, Christophers Pubns. Inc., Springville, 1991.

Coffin, Albert, *A Botanic Guide to Health*, London, 1866.

Conrow & Hecksel, *Herbal Pathfinders: Voices of the Herb Renaissance*, Woodbridge Press, Santa Barbara, 1983.

Day, Ivan, *Perfumery with Herbs*, Darton, Longman & Todd, London, UK, 1979.

de Bray, Lys, *The Wild Garden: An illustrated Guide to Weeds*, Mayflower Books, New York, 1978.

Dioscorides, *De Materia Medica*, ed. R T Gunther, Oxford University Press, 1934.

Duke, James, A., *The Green Pharmacy*, St Martin's Paperback, St Martin's Press, New York, NY100100, USA, 1997.

Duke, James, A., *Handbook of Edible Weeds*, Boca Raton, CRC Press, 1992.

Duke, James, A., *Handbook of Medicinal Herbs*, CRC Press Boca Raton, FL:CRC Press, 1985.

Fettner, Ann Tucker, *Potpourri, Incense and other Fragrant Concoctions*, Workman Publishing Co., New York, 1977.

Fluck, Hans, *Medicinal Plants: An Authentic Guide to Natural Remedies*, Avery Pub. Group, Garden City Park, 1988.

Foster, Steven, *Echinacea, Nature's Immune Enhancer*, Healing Arts Press, Rochester, Vermont, 1991.

Foster, Steven, *Herbal Bounty*, Gibbs M. Smith/Peregrine Smith Books, Salt Lake City, Utah, 1984.

Foster/Chongxi, *Herbal Emissaries: Bringing Chinese Herbs to the West*, Inner Traditions, Rochester, 1992.

Frawley, David, *Ayurvedic Healing*, Passage Press, Salt Lake City, 1989.

Frawley, David, *The Yoga of Herbs: An Ayurvedic Guide to Herbal Medicine*, Lotus Press, Santa Fe, 1988.

Fulder & Blackwood, *Garlic: Nature's Original Remedy*, Rochester, Inner Traditions, 1991.

Gerard, John, *The Herball or Generall Historie of Plantes*, John Norton, London, 1597.

Gosling, Nalda, *Successful Herbal Remedies*, Thorsons, San Francisco, 1985.

Gouzil, Dezerina, *Mother Nature's Herbs and Teas*, Oliver Press, Willits, Calif., 1975.

Graham, Judy, *Evening Primrose Oil, Inner Traditions*, Rochester, 1984.

Green, James, *Male Herbal*, Crossing Press, Freedom, 1991.

Grieve, Mrs M., *A Modern Herbal, volumes I and II*. Dover Publications, New York, 1971.

Griggs, Barbara, *Green Pharmacy*, Norman & Hobhouse, UK, 1981.

Hall, Dorothy, *Dorothy Hall's Herbal Medicine*, Thomas C. Lothian Pty Ltd, Victoria, Australia, 1988.

Hancock, Ken, *Feverfew: Your Headache may be Over*, Keats Publishing, New Cannaan, Conn., 1986.

Harrar, Sari, and O'Donnell, Sara Altshul, *The Woman's Book of Healing Herbs*, Rodale Press Inc, Emmaus, Pennsylvania, USA, 1998.

Harrer, G. and Sommer, H., 'Treatment of Mild/Moderate Depression with Hypericum', *Phytomed*, 1, 3-8, 1994.

Hills, Lawrence D., *Comfrey: Fodder, Food and Remedy*, New York, Universe Books, 1976.

Hills, Lawrence D., *Comfrey the Herbal Healer*, Bocking, Braintree, Essex, England, Henry Doubleday Research Association, n.d.

Hills, Lawrence D., *Comfrey Report: The Story of the World's Fastest Protein Builder, Bocking*, Braintree, Essex, England, Henry Doubleday Research Association, 1974.

Hobbs, C., *The Echinacea Handbook*, Eclectic Medical Publications, Portland, OR, 1989.

Hobbs, Christopher, *Foundations of Health: The Liver and Digestion Herbal*, Botanica Press, Capitola, 1992.

Hobbs, Christopher, *Ginkgo: Elixir of Youth*, Botanica Press, Capitola, 1991.

Hobbs, Christopher, *Milk Thistle: The Liver Herb*, Native Herb Co., Capitola, Calif., 1984.

Hoffmann, David, *The Elements of Herbalism*, Element Books, Shaftesbury, Dorset, 1990.

Hoffman, David, *The New Holistic Herbal*, Element Books, Shaftesbury, Dorset, 1983.

Hornsey-Pennell, Paul, *Aloe Vera The Natural Healer*, The Wordsmith Publishing Company, Bordon, Hampshire, UK, 1996.

Houdret, Jessica, *The Home Apothecary*, Lorenz Books, Anness Publishing, London, 1998.

Jacobs, Betty E. M., *Growing and Using Herbs Successfully*, Charlotte, Vt. Garden Way Publishing, 1981.

Kaptehuck, Ted, *Chinese Medicine – the Web that has no Weaver*, Rider, London, 1983.

Kartnig, T., 'Clinical Applications of Centella asiatica (L.) Urb.', *Herbs Spices Med Plants*, 3l, 146-73, 1988.

Keville, Kathi, *The Illustrated Herb Encyclopedia*, BDD Promotional Book Co. Inc., New York, 1991.

Kilham, Chris, *Kava*, Park Street Press, Rochester, Vermont, USA, 1996.

Kloss, Jethro, *Back to Eden*, Lifeline Books, Riverside, CA, USA, 1973.

Kowalchik, Claire, and Hilton, William H., eds, *Rodale's Illustrated Encyclopedia of Herbs*, Rodale Press, Emmaus, Pennsylvania, USA, 1998.

Lad, Dr V. and Frawley, D., *The Yoga of Herbs*, Lotus Press, New Mexico, 1986.

Lebot V., Merlin M., and Lindstrom L., *Kava: The Pacific Drug*, Yale University Press, New Haven, CT, 1992.

Lehane, Brendan, T*he Power of Plants*, Hohn Murray, London, 1977.

Le Strange, Richard, *A History of Herbal Plants*, New York, John Wiley & Sons, 1977.

Lu, Henry C., *Chinese System of Food Cures*, Sterling, New York, 1986.

Lust, John, *Herb Book*, Bantam Books, New York, 1982.

Mabey, Richard, *The Complete New Herbal*, Elm Tree Books, London, UK, 1988.

Mabey, Richard, *The New Age Herbalist*, Macmillan, New York, 1988.

Manniche, Lise, *An Ancient Egyptian Herbal*, British Museum Publications, London, 1989.

McIntyre, Anne, *The Complete Floral Healer*, Hodder Headline Australia Pty Ltd, Rydalmere, NSW, Australia, 1996.

McIntyre, Anne, *The Complete Woman's Herbal*, Gaia Books Ltd, London, 1994.

McIntyre, Anne, *The Herbal for Pregnancy and Childbirth*, Element Books, Shaftesbury, 1992.

McIntyre, Anne, *Herbs for Mother and Child*, Sheldon Press, London, 1988.

McIntyre, Anne, *Herbal Medicine for Everyone*, Viking Penguin, New York, 1989.

Messegue, M., *Maurice Messegue's Way to Natural Health and Beauty*, George Allen & Unwin, 1976.

Meyer, H.J., 'Pharmacology of Karva', *Ethnopharmacological Search for Psychoactive Drugs* (Holmstedt B., and Kline N.S., eds.), pp. 133-140, Raven Press, New York, 1979.

Mills, Simon, *Alternatives in Healing*, Marshall Editions, London, 1988.

Mills, Simon, *The Dictionary of Modern Herbalism: A Comprehensive Guide to Practical Herbal Therapy*, New York, Thorsons Publishers, 1985.

Mills, Simon, *Out of the Earth: The Science and Practice of Herbal Medicine*, Viking Penguin, New York, 1992.

Moerman, Daniel E., *Medicinal Plants of North America*, University of Michigan, Museum of Anthropology.

Moring, Stephen E., *Echinacea: A Natural Immune Stimulant and Treatment for Viral Infection*, Sunnyvale, Calif., Botica Analyticum, 1984.

Mowrey, Daniel, *Next Generation Herbal Medicine: Guaranteed Potency Herbs*, Keats Pubns., New Canaan, 1990.

Murray, Michael T., *The Healing Power of Herbs*, Prima Publishing, Rocklin, CA, USA, 1995.

Ody, Penelope, *The Complete Medicinal Herbal*, Dorling Kindersley, London, 1995.

Paracelsus, *Paracelsus – Selected Writings*, ed. Jolande Jacobi, Princeton University Press, 1988.

Phillips, A. and Rakusen, J., *Our Bodies, Ourselves*, Penguin Books Ltd., Harmondsworth, Middlesex, UK, 1978.

Pizzorno, Joseph E., N.D., and Murray, Michael T., N.D., *A Textbook of Natural Medicine*, John Bastyr Publications, Seattle, USA, 1987.

Pliny, *Natural History*, Harvard University Press, 1956.

Rohde, Eleanour Sinclair, *A Garden of Herbs*, P.E. Warner & Medici Society, London.

Rohde, Eleanour Sinclair, *The Old English Herbals*, Longmans, Green & Co., London, 1922.

Rose, Jeanne, *Herbs & Things*, Grosset & Dunlap, New York, USA, 1972.

Rose, Jeanne, *Jeanne Rose's Herbal Body Book*, Grosset & Dunlap, New York, USA, 1976.

Scheffer, M., *Bach Flower Therapy: Theory and Practice*, Thorsons, 1986.

Siraisi, Nancy, *Medieval and Early Renaissance Medicine*, University of Chicago Press, 1990.

St Clare, Debra, *The Herbal Medicine Chest*, Celestial Arts, Berkeley, CA, USA, 1997.

Stuart, Malcolm, ed., *The Encyclopedia of Herbs and Herbalism*, Orbis Publishing, London, 1979.

Sullivan, Dr Andrea D., *A Path to Healing*, Doubleday, New York, USA, 1998.

Svoboda, Robert E., *Ayurveda – Life Health and Longevity*, Arkana, London, 1992.

Swanson, Faith H., and Rady, Virginia B., *Herb Garden Design*, University Press of New England, Hanover, HM, 1984.

Teeguarden, Ron, *Chinese Tonic Herbs*, Japan Publications, Tokyo, 1984.

The Herbal Remedies of the Physicians of Myddfai (Meddygon Myddfai) trans. John Pughe, Llanerch Enterprises, Lampeter, 1987.

The Yellow Emperor's Classic of Internal Medicine, trans. Ilza Veith, University of California Press, 1966.

Theophrastus, *Enquiry into Plants*, 2 vols, Harvard University Press, 1916.

Thomas, Samuel, *A Narrative of the Life and Medical Discoveries of Samuel Thomson*, Boston, 1825.

Thomson, William A. R., M.D., *Herbs that Heal*, Charles Scribner's Sons, New York, 1976.

Tisserand, Robert B., *The Art of Aromatherapy*, New York, Inner Traditions International, 1979.

Turner, William, *A New Herbal, 1551*. Facsimile ed. George Chapman and Marilyn Tweddle, Carcanet Press, 1989.

Vogel, Virgil, *American Indian Medicine*, Universtiy of Oklahoma Press, 1970.

Woodward, Marcus, *Leaves from Gerad's Herball*, Houghton Mifflin, Boston, 1931.

Worwood, V, *The Fragrant Pharmacy*, Bantam Books, London, UK, 1991.

index

Page numbers in *italic* refer to the illustrations

acknowledgments

There are many people over the years who have been my teachers – far too many to list them all. I would, however, like to express special thanks to Dr Gordon Latto, Dr Barbara Latto, Dr Dagmar Leichti von Brasch, Dr Philip Kilsby, Dr Peter Mansfield, and my maternal grandmother, Yvonne Kilpatrick, who first introduced me to the power of plants. She was a fine healer and a woman of such personal power that any problem a healing plant couldn't clear, her will would finish off. I would also like to thank Priscilla Palmer at Willow Tree Herb Garden for sharing with me her passion for plants, her recipes for beauty, and some wonderful days in the sun photographing; Peter Butler at Forest Herb Research in Golden Bay whose persistent research into the power of plants brings healing to many; Gillian Poulson for sharing the beauty of her herb garden in Akaroa; and Oraina Jones for her wisdom about flower essences, her lovely Earth Song garden and the sparkle in her Elderflower Champagne.

Thanks also go to Amelia Thorpe for her doggedly insisting that I write this book long enough that I finally woke up and saw the light; to Denise Bates for her willingness to honour my vision and do everything she could to bring it into form; to Emma Callery for the hours that she has spent wrestling with my spelling; to Brenda Thard my teacher in nature photography, and to the Maine Photographic Workshops for making it possible for me to learn from her; to Keith Wynn for holding my hand while I eased my way into macro photography at times when he had 10,000 other things to do.

I am enormously grateful for the talent, skill and passion that the book's designer, Ruth Prentice, has put into the project – spending many hours with me in front of an Apple Mac screen manipulating double-page spreads. As ever this book would not have been written at all had it not been for the endless hard work put in to helping me produce it by my best friend and help-mate, The Fox. Finally, and most important of all, I want to thank the spirits of the wonderful plants who shared with me their wisdom, their humour, their vibrant life-force, and their love – from the shy viola to the rampant and wicked poppy.